LIVING
WITH
TERMINAL
LUNG
CANCER

A STORY OF HOPE

Also by William Schuette

White Blaze Fever

LIVING WITH TERMINAL LUNG CANCER

A STORY OF HOPE

WILLIAM
SCHUETTE

Published by *WGS*

ISBN NUMBER

ISBN 979-8-9880630-1-8 (Soft Bound)

ISBN 979-8-9880630-0-1 (Hard Cover)

ISBN 979-8-9880630-2-5 (e-book)

Book Cover and Interior Formatting by 100 Covers

Dedication

To my wife Connie, without whom this book would never have made it to press. Her support and encouragement were paramount from inception to the finish line.

Foreword

Have you ever been desperate for hope? *Living with Terminal Lung Cancer* is a remarkable journey of hope; taking the reader on an emotional roller coaster ride from diagnosis to the front lines of the battlefield. A must-read for anyone who has ever heard the words cancer or terminal. It is a literal roadmap of what can happen when love, the will to live, and medical research collide.

This is a story of one man's journey of how lack of educational awareness about lung cancer in the medical community delayed his diagnosis and exposed him to unnecessary treatments, culminating ultimately in sending him home to die. But he is still *Living with Terminal Lung Cancer*; 16 years later!

When my husband Jeff was diagnosed with terminal lung cancer in 2015, given less than a year to live, we were desperate for hope. In my search, I discovered Bill and his wife, Connie, living in a small rural Ohio town 20 miles from us. How is it possible he is still alive and traveling the world eight years after his diagnosis? Nothing could give us more hope than to see what is possible, face to face; if he can live with lung cancer, so can we. Even today, eight years later, witnessing their journey is an invaluable silver lining to our journey with cancer.

It is my hope every reader will learn it is possible to live with terminal lung cancer and how the lack of awareness about this disease has placed great burdens on those impacted by lung cancer to navigate access to appropriate testing and treatments. Public health campaigns have only taught one risk factor for developing lung cancer, tobacco addiction.

Every year more people are diagnosed with lung cancer than breast, colon, and prostate combined; many of those have never suffered from tobacco addiction. Did you know environmental exposures such as radon are the second leading cause of lung cancer? Why is this important? The unintended consequences of this lack of awareness are life and death.

While Bill's journey highlights advancements in lung cancer testing and treatments, modern research, testing, and treatments are useless if they are not utilized! It is important for the reader to recognize the main reason why Bill is still living with terminal lung cancer; 16 years after being told he would not be alive in a year. Quite simply, Bill never gave up hope; with his wife Connie by his side, they show us the power of being your own healthcare advocate. From his death bed, Bill still had a fierce will to live; the journey from rural Ohio to Boston is mind-blowing and a testament to the importance of awareness, self-advocacy, and sharing our journeys.

—Rhonda Meckstroth
Lung Cancer Advocate/Care Partner

Rhonda is an advocate for lung cancer, biomarker testing, healthcare advocacy, and care partners. She is an administrator for a large worldwide ALK Positive Lung Cancer Support Group; is a Board Member for the White Ribbon Project; and also works with pharmaceutical companies, researchers, medical professionals, and advocacy organizations such as the National Lung Cancer Roundtable, Lung Cancer Research Foundation, International Association for the Study of Lung Cancer, and the Caregiver Action Network.

"One day you will tell your story of how you overcame what you went through and it will be someone else's survival guide." —Berne Brown

Preface

I share the following "morsels of wisdom" with no illusion that I am a scholar or superior to anyone who reads this book. Instead, I am an authority on the aspects of surviving and living with cancer by default only; in other words, I have become knowledgeable not by desire but simply by need!

I am a stage IV lung cancer survivor about to share a journey of *"Living with Terminal Lung Cancer."* A journey that, in a span of sixteen years, has had many highs and lows that at times seemed unconquerable; yet with the help of a steadfast wife/caretaker and a remarkable oncologist, I have persevered. My cancer journey has been both a marathon and a sprint, sometimes leaving me breathless with pain and despair while other times with hope and solace. I have endeavored to bring my journey to the reader firsthand through the eyes of a person living with cancer, conveying my thoughts and reactions as the events of cancer infiltrated my life.

While each person living with cancer is unique because of their particular cancer, there are constants; similarities, if you will. When diagnosed, each patient will have a journey before them with the highs and lows I referenced. It is my goal, as one who has been on this difficult journey for 16 years, to assist patients recently diagnosed, along with caregivers, family, and friends, through suggestions and examples via my experience.

It is my sincere intent to comfort patients recently diagnosed with cancer to know that there is hope, my years of survival being a real testament. The advent of new drugs like TKI's (Tyrosine Kinase Inhibitor) and immunotherapies being developed in the labs by very conscientious scientists daily, many in clinical trials, has bolstered the potential to increase the chance for survival, along with providing the all-important quality of life. Currently, biomarker testing and liquid biopsies are game changers for lung cancer survivor rates.

I have a story, actually many stories, to let my readers know there is hope for a person living with cancer. I am living proof; I am a 16-year cancer survivor!

Acknowledgments

I would like to thank Linda Moody, Carol Hemmerich, and Tom Donnelly for their advice, encouragement, and editorial assistance.

A special acknowledgment to

Dr. Alice Shaw, M.D., Ph.D.

and

Rhonda Meckstroth ALK-Positive Support Group Adm.

"I won't let cancer define me, but I'll use my journey to help others." —Doug Clark

Introduction

Newly diagnosed patients have a difficult journey ahead of them with many obstacles and challenges. The reader will find in my book, *"Living with Terminal Lung Cancer"*, a candid insight into my cancer journey, along with suggestions to assist with the obstacles and challenges of cancer.

Examples and insights are intended not only for the patient but also for the caregiver, family, and friends. Who are critical and invaluable assets in the patient's lung cancer journey as they live with this disease. Note, I call it a journey, for that, is what it simply is, an extension of one's life journey.

Throughout *"Living with Terminal Lung Cancer"*, I have incorporated basic examples of what a person living with cancer and his caregiver and friends need to consider to not only survive cancer but to enjoy a good quality of life. I share through my travels how a terminal lung cancer survivor can safely travel, be it the world or our beautiful United States of America. Interspersed throughout my book, the reader will find pictures of places traveled, friends, and family, illustrating my belief in living with lung cancer. I share this information as it happened to me, and hopefully, you, the reader, will avoid some of the pitfalls I encountered while finding enlightenment in my positive experience. A must-read for all individuals living with cancer and caregivers, including information specific to ALK-positive lung cancer.

Contents

*"Cancer is only going to be a chapter in your life,
not the whole story."* —Joe Wasser

Prologue

2007 – Cleveland Clinic – Family Conference with Oncologist

**"You have Adenocarcinoma non-small cell lung cancer", a
very solemn and expressionless doctor continued, "Stage IV;
it's terminal."**

The diagnosis hit me like a fist in the gut. I and my wife and three
adult children sat in the tiny sterile hospital room that seemed to
shrink and close in on me as we listened to the oncologist's diagnosis. My eyes shifted from child to child and then to my wife; their
looks of disbelief screamed out at me.

My mind raced. How could this be? I never smoked. All the
doctors told me how great my health was. It wasn't but a few
months earlier, I had been competing in Senior Olympic Triath-
lons, for God's sake! Now they were telling me I had six months to
two years to live! How could this be?

*"There's a commonly held perception that 'they did
it to themselves' or that all lung cancer is caused by
tobacco use. In reality, the only risk factor for getting
lung cancer is having lungs."*
—Dr. Stephanie Snow
President of Lung Cancer Canada

It may be best if I start at the beginning.

CHAPTER 1
A Cancer Diagnosis

*"When you are diagnosed, surround yourself with
the best medical providers and uplifting friends.
Going through cancer is scary and you can easily go down
a path of negativity and darkness. But you can't let yourself
do that. You need to have positivity and encouragement
from others. It truly does help you through your healing."*
—Charlotte Shaff

* * * * * * * * *

For a year or so, I had been feeling discomfort in my chest. Ever so faint in the beginning, as time passed, the puzzling discomfort seemed to increase in severity. Yet, yearly physicals with my doctor always gave me a clean bill of health. Obviously, good health was what I wanted to hear, so I continued to push the discomfort issue into the recesses of my mind.

My wife never liked me describing my chest pain as a discomfort, feeling that calling the pain only a discomfort minimized the symptoms, thus encouraging the attending physician to ignore a more serious problem. But to me, that's what it was, just a minor discomfort, at least early on.

Although apparently in excellent shape for my age, fifty-eight. I had shared my concern with various doctors about my chest discomfort and how it seemed more intense with time. Hearing that my mother died of a heart attack at the young age of fifty-one, my family physician thought it prudent to have an EKG and chest X-ray in his office. The chest X-ray proved negative; overall, the EKG results looked good except for a slight blip on the printout. Because of the blip issue, my doctor scheduled a stress test at the local hospital.

I believe it was around this time I asked my doctor if the pain I was experiencing could be related to anything like cancer. I don't know why I thought I had cancer. Possibly it was related to the fact that a very close friend, my same-aged cousin, had died from esophageal cancer earlier, and it was still on my mind. His response was rather quick and dismissive, something along the lines that I was not a smoker, in very good shape, and had no family history of lung cancer; therefore, the probability of me having lung cancer was minimal. He sounded confident, and again I put it away; I was looking for that type of reassurance.

As anticipated, I basically "blew the lid" off the stress test at the hospital. Besides the irregular EKG blip, I was in excellent shape, or so we all thought. After reviewing the results, the doctor recommended carrying on as I had been but monitoring the "chest discomfort" and be prepared for more elaborate tests if the pain continued or increased. It was about this time my wife and I had planned to take a Mediterranean cruise. When I shared this with the doctor, he reiterated that I should continue my typical plans and monitor my chest pain.

As the days passed, the chest pains continued, with a noticeable increase in intensity. Not sure if this increase in pain was due to a more severe problem, a chest cold, or just anxiety about traveling overseas, I began to have doubts about the wisdom of such a trip.

Having worked as a bicycle guide overseas for a time, I had the very memorable experience of observing two clients race down a mountainside in Greece with the spirit of "Lance Armstrong," only to result in a horrifying over-the-handle-bars flight ending with a face-first landing on a very unforgiving gravel/asphalt pavement! Their fall ended with some very nasty road rash, not to mention bruised egos and a trip to the hospital.

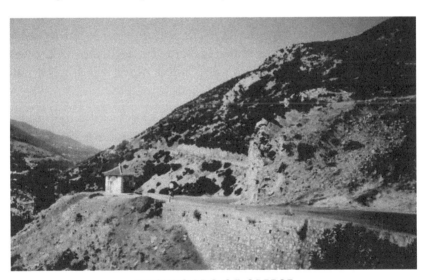

BACKROADS OF GREECE

After the arrival and delivery of the injured riders to the hospital medical staff, I promptly sought out a restroom to wash my hands. Opening the door, I was immediately shocked by the uncleanliness of the facility. Particularly repulsive were the sight and smell of a soiled diaper lying in the corner of the room.

Later, with the medical staff's approval to obtain the x-ray copies of my two bruised and battered riders, my negativity only escalated when entering the x-ray room. Upon opening the door, I was blasted by thick smoke that literally took my breath away. As I squinted my eyes and waved a hand to clear the dense smoke, the slight glow of what seemed to be two cigarettes began to speak.

"Can we help you?" I finally realized that the two glowing cigarettes actually belonged to two x-ray technicians on a smoke break! Still waving my hand to clear away the smoke, I sheepishly apologized for interrupting their smoke break and shared that I was told I could obtain copies of the riders' x-rays. "Sure. Not a problem," was the response of one tech, who then walked over to the screen, ripped off the x-rays, and handed them to me. When I asked about payment, he smiled, opened the door to let me out, and said, "No charge. Have a great day."

What remained ingrained in my mind during the hospital visit was a very negative experience. Consequently, I went away with a questionable opinion of their socialized medicine. Therefore, I knew a Mediterranean cruise was not a place I wanted to be if indeed, I was having severe heart issues.

Over the next few days at home, my chest pains increased to the point that I ended up in the hospital ER, where another EKG was performed. The continued blip results led the attending physician to recommend a transfer to the Dayton Heart Hospital for a heart catheterization. After a bit of embarrassment that nothing abnormal was found and an overnight stay in the hospital, the heart doctors gave me a clean bill of health.

Although relieved to know my heart was healthy and strong, the chest pain continued, and although not debilitating to any extent, I just "KNEW" something was not right. On a follow-up trip to my family doctor, we discussed the excellent heart catheterization results, but still no answer for the continued chest discomfort.

The doc admitted he was stumped and suggested I see a pulmonary specialist for further testing. He also asked me to consider a colonoscopy, implying that it would be prudent if I had not had one, especially since we were no closer to knowing what was causing the chest pain. He also prescribed an antibiotic along with aspirin. It was obvious to me that we were indeed grasping for straws as 2006 came to an end.

A colonoscopy was scheduled, and the attending physician told me my colon was clear and looked very healthy after the procedure. Noticing the perplexed look on my face, he asked if there was anything else he could do for me. Detecting a glimmer of hope, without hesitation, I said, "yes." After sharing my concern over not knowing what was causing my chest pain, I asked about the possibility of a chest X-ray just to help me rest a little easier. To my surprise, he said "sure" and wheeled in an X-ray machine and had the X-ray done immediately.

Later, my family physician shared the clean colonoscopy and chest X-ray report, changed my antibiotics, prescribed a medicated inhaler, and scheduled a visit to the pulmonologist. The positive results made me feel a little better, yet the deep nagging chest pain continued.

As I entered the waiting room of the pulmonary specialist, I felt very out of place. With tanks, tubes, and wheelchairs all over the place, it seemed everyone in the waiting room had sad, forlorn eyes and some type of breathing apparatus coming out of their nose. To be honest, I was entirely disheartened and unsettled by the experience.

The uncomfortable, awkward feeling did not dissipate as I talked with the pulmonologist, for I could tell from his questions he was really wondering what I was doing in his office. As I described a discomfort when breathing deeply, his body language matched his questions. But to ease my mind, he said he would schedule a Pulmonary Function and a Methacholine Challenge test with a follow-up visit.

For the follow-up visit, I invited my wife to accompany me and hear first-hand how lackadaisical the specialist was about my chest pain concerns. While I was hearing what I wanted to hear, that there was nothing wrong with me, I really began to be annoyed by the casual, indifferent attitude of the pulmonologist. After completing the test, it was no surprise that I had performed very well, and I figured this would fuel his lax attitude. It did, but I was totally taken aback by his, let me call it, delivery of diagnosis as he exploded into the exam room and exclaimed very distinctly and boldly, "You are disease-free!"

He continued, with the look of a disgruntled parent talking with his child, by saying most patients in his office would give anything to have my lungs. He then suggested some breathing medicine, almost as a second thought, reassuring me that he had seen this condition many times and there was no reason to be overly concerned. He finished by saying, in passing, he would see me in six months.

That was all I needed to hear. I had had enough waiting and uncertainty. Six months was entirely too long, and not wanting to wait another half year, I asked the doctor if he could possibly arrange for me to have a CT scan. Showing a total lack of concern, he smiled and, shaking his head, said something to the effect that a CT scan was way down the road. Thus, I left his office with a prescription in hand for an inhaler and a follow-up visit in six months if the discomfort did not abate. His comments and body language left little doubt that he was very confident he would never see me again.

Out in the parking lot, my wife and I looked at each other in total bewilderment and asked, "Where do we go now?" It was becoming painfully evident that I would have to become my own advocate. The answers to my chest pain would not be dropped off at my doorstep; I would have to find the answer on my own.

Needless to say, the inhaler did not work. Nothing had changed, and I was still experiencing chest pain when breathing deeply. Even with all the positive feedback from tests and doctors and wanting to believe their reports, I knew deep down inside that my body was telling me something was wrong. I was determined to get to the bottom of it, but I was unsure how. I was totally frustrated with not knowing what to do next.

*****

As luck would have it, a month later, as I was mulling over my situation at home, I came across a newspaper advertisement for a CT screening. The screening was for smokers but available to anyone; although I had never smoked, I thought this would put to bed any thoughts I had in the back of my mind about cancer. What really caught my eye was it did not require a physician's order. I thought this was what I needed; although my health insurance did not cover it and my wallet would be a little lighter, the cost was only one hundred dollars. It would be an inexpensive "peace of mind."

So, on our way south from Ohio for a planned trip to Florida, my wife and I made a quick side trip west on I-70 to the Richmond, Indiana, Reid Memorial Hospital for a quick "smokers" CT screening. And quick it was; I didn't even have to take my shirt off and literally was out of the CT screening room before my wife had a chance to turn the first page in her *Better Homes & Gardens* magazine. A swipe of the credit card for one hundred dollars and three minutes later, we were on the road to sunny Florida without a care in the world. Little could I imagine how my life was about to be turned inside out.

Chapter 2
You Have a Problem

*"I learned a long time ago the wisest thing I can do
is be on my own side, be an advocate
for myself and others like me."*
—Maya Angelou

* * * * * * * *

A week later, after a pleasant and relaxing visit with friends in Florida, we stopped at a roadside rest to check phone messages at home. And so, the nightmare began.

I received a voice message from a nurse in my family physician's office to give them a call. Although a little apprehensive about getting a call from my physician, I was not prepared for what I was about to hear. The receptionist immediately put the doctor on the phone and his first comment was, "Bill, who sent you for a CT in Richmond?" Caught off guard with such an abrupt question, I responded, "Why, no one." I continued a bit coarsely that the pulmonary specialist he had sent me to had been no help and that I felt the specialist did not take my concerns seriously, telling me to see him in six months.

I continued, "Frankly, I found the pulmonologist condescending and too dismissive for my liking." I finished by saying that my displeasure with the pulmonologist led me to take matters into my own hands, and I went for a CT screening on my own. The phone went dead silent, and although probably just seconds, it seemed like an eternity until from the other end of the phone came, "Bill, you've got a problem."

The rest of our conversation was a blur, but I do remember him saying I had what appeared to be lung cancer, and it seemed to have metastasized. I remember mumbling something ridiculous like, "This is serious," and his, "Yes, it is." My mind raced with a mixture of unanswered questions and disbelief as I ended the call and turned to my wife with a look of total bewilderment.

She had been listening to everything on speaker phone and we just stared at each other in absolute shock. I had just been told I had a metastasized form of lung cancer, and although ignorant of exactly what that meant, the term "metastasized cancer" sent chills down my backbone.

* * * * *

One thousand miles from home, in the parking lot of a Georgia roadside rest, I had been given a death sentence by my doctor. Now what?

Not at all sure of what to do or where to go next, I did know there would be no more local doctors in the equation. I was angry. My mind screamed, "I told you something was wrong!" For months; no, years! I had been seeking answers to no avail, and now they tell me I had metastasized lung cancer. I really wanted to go and beat the hell out of someone!!

Numbed and shell-shocked, I'm not sure which one of us thought of her first, but my niece, a physician at the Cleveland Clinic, would be our next move. Another roadside call, this time to my sister in Cleveland, was emotional, to say the least, and to be very honest, I don't remember much. Looking back on it now, I probably should have waited awhile to compose myself before calling, but "logical thinking" was not high on my agenda, nor anything involving more waiting. Within an hour, my niece was on the phone and making arrangements for me to see a pulmonologist she knew very well at the Cleveland Clinic and for whom she had the utmost respect—seemingly a slight ray of sunlight amidst a sea of turmoil.

Upon arrival at home, I informed my family physician that I was foregoing any local doctors and had made arrangements to see a doctor at the Cleveland Clinic. Without hesitation, he agreed I had made the correct decision. I was not angry with my family physician. He had tried to find out what was causing my difficulties. Rather, I was just so frustrated that it had taken so long to find the problem. I learned later in my cancer battle that an early lung cancer diagnosis is paramount. I was particularly angry with my local pulmonologist's seemingly uncaring attitude towards my chest pain.

Looking back on the "what ifs," I believe a person with cancer must tread lightly. The "what ifs" can drive you crazy if you dwell on them. Obviously, it would have been much better if the cancer had been caught at an early stage, but the fact remains that we did not catch it early on, and I now needed to deal with the "here and now."

Within a few days, I was sitting in the office of another pulmonologist at the Cleveland Clinic discussing a bronchoscopy biopsy and PET scan. He shared that I had cause for concern, but a biopsy would be needed to determine precisely what we were looking at and our next move. In an attempt to cover all possibilities, and I believe to ease my concern, he stated that a CT scan often could show scars or images that may or may not be cancerous. There was even a particular fungus occasionally found in the lungs in our part of the Ohio Midwest that often was not cancerous. Although a bit relieved by the different possibilities, I continued to be extremely distraught, to say the least.

The doctor ordered a bronchoscopy biopsy, and I was told the procedure had its challenges. The tumor they hoped to biopsy was relatively small, near a blood vessel and my heart. Ideally, they could reach it through my windpipe. If not, they would need to run a needle through my chest, not something they or I desired.

After the procedure, the doctor met with me and shared that all had gone well. They were able to get a sample on their first try. Of particular interest, the doctor conveyed he felt good about the biopsy, but tests on the sample would have to be completed, and he would call me with the results. The following day I had a PET scan. Although I did not know any results, the doctor's positive demeanor made me feel pretty good on my drive home, and I looked forward to the first good night's sleep in days and a call, hopefully telling me everything was OK.

* * * * *

Over the weekend, I anxiously awaited hearing that the biopsy was not cancer. On April 8, 2007, the doctor's phone call finally came in and again brought my world crashing down as he shared that the biopsy test was positive for Adenocarcinoma, non-small cell lung cancer. My heart sank. So here it was; I had lung cancer. My life, what was left of it, would be changed forever. The doctor assured me he would connect me with an outstanding oncologist at the Cleveland Clinic. The slight ray of hope was all but the flicker of a candle by this time.

Back in Cleveland, my wife and I went for a detailed look at what was growing in my chest and, more importantly, my options. My children flew in from New York, Virginia, and California. I had not given them much information, not wanting to worry them needlessly. There would be no "sugar coating" now; the time had come for us to learn precisely what I had and what I could expect.

Fortunately, my sister lived in Cleveland and offered to have us all stay at her home in preparation for the conference with the oncologist. Not having to worry about making arrangements for myself and the children was of great comfort. My sister's thoughtfulness and caring have never ceased; she has been the consummate protective sister to this day.

As time passed, family and friends continued to be even more special. I have learned a great deal about family, friends, and others. As a person living with cancer, when you are genuinely in need, the very caring help in any way possible. However, sadly, there are those few who just want to know enough to pass on gossip.

After the initial shock of hearing from the oncologist that my lung cancer was stage IV and terminal, my first thought was, OK, now what? My ignorance was apparent and was immediately met with a very negative, nothing-you-can-do attitude by the doctor. His so-called "bedside manner" was not what I had expected. Trying to be fair, I surmised that the doctor probably dealt with cancer every day and naturally would have become callous to the disease, but his matter-of-fact attitude was a bit over the top.

With the information mentioned above, one would think it was "all over" for the recipient of that kind of "smash mouth" talk from a doctor. I had asked for it straight, but to be very honest, I had not expected the answer to be that harsh.

When hit with such a hellish diagnosis, I reacted like most and immediately asked naively what treatment options I would be looking at? The response from the very callous oncologist was nothing more than devastating when he told me that stage IV NSCLC meant no surgery, no radiation, just chemo, and, did I mention, no cure? As I learned later, this oncologist was uninformed about the latest cancer science and treatments.

He was so defeatist and downright arrogant that my youngest son sitting in on the conference simply got up and left. This seemed to irritate the doctor as he immediately directed his assistant, who had been sitting in on the conference, to return my son to the room. I suggested that would not be necessary, figuring my son needed a little space and time. The doctor basically blew off my comment and, with an apparent need for control, sent his assistant out to bring my son back. Knowing my son, I knew this was not the best thing to do; however, it was obvious by this time that this doctor was not one to be told what to do. It wasn't but a couple of minutes later the assistant was back in the room with a "deer in the headlights" look on his face saying something to the effect that "everything's cool!" I must admit a slight smile crossed my face knowing my youngest son had had enough and probably let the assistant know his feelings in no uncertain terms. To be perfectly honest, I was a bit surprised to see the young assistant return at all. Knowing my son, he could just as easily be sitting in the Cleveland Clinic surgery nursing a very distorted nose!

I probably should have thanked the doctor then and there and immediately began searching for a second opinion, exiting as fast as I had entered! However, this was all new to me, and I was unprepared to make such an aggressive move. Looking back on the years interacting with cancer and doctors, I certainly would have requested a change. I believe it is called "Being Your Own Advocate," a must motto for all those living with cancers.

Our conference continued with me asking about options. I was told very matter-of-factly that the only option was some form of chemotherapy but that it was not likely to be very effective. With my limited knowledge of cancer and the different treatments, my mind raced as it tried to get some positive direction.

"What about radiation?" I asked. "No, not possible; the cancer is too widespread. That's why it is stage IV," was the flat response. I'm scrambling by now, "What about surgery?" I asked. Same answer, "Cancer is too widespread."

About this time, it got very quiet; my oldest son broke the silence with a question. I don't even remember what it was, but it was answered with the same negative response.

Again quiet, the hopelessness was deafening. The oncologist finally broke the silence, "We need to think outside the box." I'll never forget this statement. For a moment, I thought that now we were getting somewhere! This sense of elation did not last long; the doctor began discussing the possibility of me qualifying for a phase II clinical trial they were starting at the Clinic.

A clinical trial? I thought. Let me assure you, this definitely did not fit my definition of thinking "outside the box." I was still looking for some type of surgery/radiation that would remove the disease from my body! Disappointed, I listened as the doctor discussed the clinical trial, what to expect, procedures, timeline, cost, etc. All this led to my final question, which I knew was on the mind of everyone in the room, "How long do I have?" Without hesitation and any uncertainty, "Six months to two years, depending on the effectiveness of the chemo" was his very casual response.

I had heard enough. I needed some time to digest this devastating news. While respecting the doctor's diagnosis, I shared that I wanted a second opinion. He seemingly understood and agreed that a second opinion was warranted, thus bringing our somewhat contentious meeting to a close. Feeling that so much time had been wasted, I felt an urgency to get started and wondered out loud if delaying the chemo until I talked with another doctor would be detrimental. Continuing the negativity, the doctor stated with an air of hopelessness that there was no urgency, reiterating that my stage IV diagnosis was terminal.

* * * * *

Over a somber lunch at my sister's home, my family sat down and put our heads together to secure a doctor for a second opinion. Some previous leg work by my daughter expedited the search. She had received the name of a well-known oncologist at Memorial Sloan-Kettering Cancer Center in New York. A visit to a New York doctor for a second opinion was precisely what my New York City resident daughter wanted to hear. Needless to say, she was not happy with what we had heard in Cleveland and did not like the negativity from the oncologist.

Still, a little stung by the lack of sensitivity and the creativity from our conference with the oncologist, I nevertheless sought out his opinion on the merits of the oncologist we were considering for a second opinion. He commented that he knew the NY doctor and highly approved of our choice. The afternoon was spent making phone calls to the New York hospital, securing an appointment, completing faxed forms, and finally talking with the Cleveland Clinic about sending biopsy samples to NY.

I later read that asking the attending physician for a recommendation was probably not the best way of selecting a physician for a second opinion. They typically refer a friend who may not want to upset their friendship with a differing opinion. Fortunately for me, looking back now, the referred physician turned out to be very knowledgeable, open and sensitive to my extremely precarious condition.

So, with forms completed, appointments scheduled, and confirmed with the hope of a fresh new look at my cancer, I was back in the car and on a trip to New York. Little did I know that hopping in the car and heading east would become a familiar part of my life as I drove the very bumpy road of cancer.

Even though he basically gave me the same diagnosis, the Sloan Kettering doctor was much more attuned to me and my family's feelings to the point of taking the extra step of asking if I had actually seen the CT scan of my cancer. When I shared that I had not, he immediately took me to the scan room, pointed out my cancer and explained thoroughly why the different options I had asked about were not feasible at the present time. It was a seemingly small action, but I assure you, it was something I appreciated and needed at the time.

While much more comfortable with the explanation and caring style of the oncologist, the fact remained I had stage IV lung cancer. At this time, very little could be done besides the relatively ineffective chemotherapy. I particularly remember the ride from his office with my wife and daughter down the elevator afterward. It was very quiet, and I was one whipped, depressed soul fighting back the tears.

That was a first. I could not remember ever tearing up in front of my daughter. While somewhat embarrassed, I would come to learn in the coming months and years of my cancer journey that, sadly, tears would be a part of the baggage on that journey. Tears were a strange phenomenon for me, for I had always viewed tears as a weakness; men don't cry. But I'll be damned if I didn't find myself with moist eyes on numerous occasions throughout my cancer journey. A whole new experience, for never before had I exhibited that type of raw emotion; yet thinking back, I guess I had never dealt with cancer and death on such a personal level.

Chapter 3
Cancer Treatments

"There are so many people out there who will tell you that you can't. What you've got to do is turn around and say 'Watch me.'"

—Author Unknown

* * * * * * * *

The obvious option, the only option, was to return to the Cleveland Clinic and begin the Phase II Clinical Trial. Little did I know the misery that lay before me. Please note: in no way is my negativity about any individual condemnation of the institution. The Cleveland Clinic is one of the finest medical facilities in the nation. I simply found the oncologist difficult to communicate with, and at the time, I did not need an adversary; I needed a positive, informed leader. Side note: I learned much later by "word of mouth" that the aforementioned oncologist is no longer there.

I returned to Cleveland with a great deal of anticipation and anxiety. After what seemed to be a long time of waiting and wondering, I had a very strong desire to finally get started. At the same time, I was very apprehensive about what to expect. I learned early on that whenever I asked about what to expect when taking chemotherapy, the reply was typical, "We don't know. It varies with each individual." That response was generally followed by an example of someone having very few negative side effects from the drug. What I was soon to find out, unfortunately, I would be one of those patients that had every negative reaction they had ever seen with the drug.

My first experience with cancer treatment, the Phase II Clinical Trial drug HKI, certainly set the stage for some very harsh reactions. At the clinic, my oncologist introduced me to the Phase II nurse practitioner for the HKI Clinical Trial, who was to guide me through the trial process. I started the clinical trial with wires hooked up to all parts of my body for an electrocardiogram and another CT scan to get a baseline. This action instigated the feeling I had heard shared by so many when entering a clinical trial, that of being the proverbial "guinea pig."

After the tests, the nurse sat down and gave me a brief rundown of what was expected of me and what I could expect from the trial. Obviously, there were no guarantees, and sadly I did not sense much optimism. I knew this going in, and I'm certainly not critical of the nurse, but "hope does spring eternal," Unfortunately, I did not have much hope at the time.

After the initial dose, I was given enough pills for one week. Six capsules to take once a day and a diary to keep track of diet, medications, and side effects. I was to return weekly for a checkup and monitoring.

It wasn't long until the side effects started to manifest themselves, and my body began early on to let me know the pills were extremely nasty. Nausea became the norm as I struggled to get the drug digested. That was followed by a terrible bout of dehydration that escalated throughout the duration of the trial. With this dehydration came the pronounced weakening and overall tearing down of my body. With the loss of strength, sleep became the norm, and in time I was so dehydrated that one visit was extended to include an IV of fluids.

After four weeks of the HKI drug, I returned to Cleveland for my scheduled checkup and first CT scan to see what, if any, changes had occurred. My oncologist brought in the CT results and shared that there was no visible change. Then the most bizarre thing happened! As the oncologist began talking about the next month on the study, to my amazement and bewilderment, he switched in midstream, saying, "No sense in beating a dead horse," and abruptly took me off the study! The comment and decision totally caught me off guard. I was stunned. At the same time, to be very honest, I was ready to end the study. I was an absolute mess, both physically and mentally.

*****

So ended my first of many negative experiences as I suffered through an "onslaught" of different cancer treatments. While I was ready to move on from the clinical trial, little did I know or could I imagine how very long and arduous the road ahead would be.

Now that the clinical trial was over, I had no idea what would be next. I had not given it much thought. Up to that day (when entering the clinical trial room), I always thought the trial would last at least a couple of months. With the trial ending so abruptly, I was at a total loss as to what would be next.

Tarceva was the call. When I asked the doctor, "why Tarceva," he stated, "We're looking for a home run." Now that got my attention! But when I asked what he considered a home run, his response of another couple of years really hit home, pardon the pun. For always in my mind, a home run was just that: a home run, a clean sweep of the bases, a clean sweep of cancer out of my body forever. Thus began the lingering thought that typically consumes all those living with cancer as they battle for their life and deal with the challenging years of cancer treatments such as chemotherapy that being "quality of life," which leads to the ultimate question, "When do I quit the fight?'

Tarceva, one of the newest drugs approved and on the market, had shown some benefits for certain lung cancers. A side note: I later learned from Dr. Alice Shaw that Tarceva only works in patients with EGFR mutations. This was known when I was treated, but testing was not widely available. EGFR mutations can be found in never-smokers, so they hoped I might respond to Tarceva since I was a never-smoker. It should be noted that smoking is not necessarily, in all cases, the primary or leading risk factor for lung cancer. This highlights the importance of molecular profiling of lung cancers and identifying the underlying target. Empiric selection (basically guessing) does NOT work! My oncologist shared that it was a rather expensive drug (it turned out to be very expensive, to the tune of ten thousand dollars a month), but financial assistance was available.

So, it was down to the hospital pharmacy to obtain the (pills) drug. Being my first experience purchasing such a costly drug, I was dismayed that my drug insurance was limited in the amount that would be paid, so the deductible was quickly reached and surpassed. Eventually, we walked out of the pharmacy with drug in hand but much, much lighter in the wallet.

In fairness to the manufacturer of Tarceva, when I called them for my second month supply of the drug, I spoke with a very personable and knowledgeable representative. He not only listened to my concerns about the high cost and out-of-pocket expenses I had already paid but directed me very quickly, I might add, through a process that enabled me to obtain the drug at little additional cost.

I have spent most of my sixteen-year journey living with lung cancer in clinical trials where the drug is typically supplied at no cost. But I have heard from others living with lung cancer and can confirm that dealing directly with the drug company is always a good place to start.

Once home and on Tarceva, my difficulties multiplied. The dehydration continued along with weakness and constant fatigue. This compounded the numerous new side effects, including a terrible rash that manifested itself when I came into contact with the sun. Special soaps, creams, and a prescription for a particular antibiotic lotion did little to stop the rash. My outdoor life of hiking and biking, which I loved, came to an abrupt end. To put it simply, I was miserable.

My only thought was that it had to get better. If not, I could handle anything for a time if indeed, the drug was working. It had been stated that a severe rash could be anticipated and possibly an indication the medication was working. This was honestly the only thought that got me through this painful, difficult time.

At the end of one month on Tarceva, another scan showed no detectable reduction of my lung cancer. It was certainly depressing news, to say the least, especially considering how lousy I had felt. In consultation with the oncologist, he recommended the addition of the chemo, Avastin, suggesting that it would be more aggressive and possibly lead to the cancer reduction we hoped to achieve. The decision was mine; was I up to a double hit of chemo?

When I started the chemo regimen, I was in pretty good shape. I had figured, admittedly somewhat presumptuously, if I were going to be taking chemotherapy I might as well take all they had to offer. And although weakened and miserable and not getting any stronger, my only thought was, bring it on!

* * * * *

Since Avastin would require an infusion and a call for much closer monitoring, it was recommended that I begin seeing an oncologist closer to my home than the two-hundred-and-fifty-mile drive to Cleveland. It was also obvious the "out of the box" oncologist was, should I say, "back in the box." To be honest, I was also ready to move on. I just didn't know to whom, how, or where to turn.

Within a week, I was seeing a new oncologist locally and beginning weekly infusions of Avastin along with my daily dose of Tarceva. The infusion process was an all-new experience for me; honestly, I did not look forward to it. I had experienced the process as an observer when I accompanied my father-in-law during his battle with pancreatic cancer and saw first-hand how tough the infusion process could be. Sitting in an oversized reclining chair with bags of drugs (I tend to call it poison) being pumped into one's body via a needle has to be one of the most difficult and depressing activities a person living with cancer endures. What I had not been privy to was the after-effect of flooding one's vein with such a potent drug. I was now about to experience it first-hand and did not relish the thought.

At the end of eight weeks, a consultation with my local oncologist, who had talked "very briefly" with my oncologist at the Cleveland Clinic (apparently, the clinic oncologist had difficulty remembering me as a patient) brought about a change. My local oncologist discontinued the Tarceva and added a new combination drug called Carboplatin/Paclitaxel. With negative visions and memories of chemotherapy treatments, I hesitated; but was knocked back to reality when my new local oncologist asked a simple question,

"What are you going to do? Just wait to die?"

That was a challenge I couldn't turn down. I gave the nod and said, "Let's do it," but believe me, there was a lump in my throat and a chill in my bones.

Now I found myself sitting for hours in the infusion room twice a week, getting what seemed like a massive dose of poison into my veins. I had said, "Give me your best shot," and they certainly were doing so. The side effects were horrendous. With the stop of Tarceva, there was some relief from the nasty, painful rash; but the loss of hair, a metallic taste to the food, continued nausea, and fatigue was absolutely overwhelming.

At the same time, I began to experience a significant drop in my white blood cell count, to the extreme degree that my infusions had to be delayed while I received shots to get back to an allowable level. The numerous injections, while raising my white blood cell count, caused a considerable amount of bone pain. I had not anticipated this amount of pain from a simple shot. Still, it was explained that the pain was not at all abnormal and actually expected—another of the many "little" surprises that accompanied chemotherapy.

A low white blood cell count meant my immune system was very low, and I was susceptible to various illnesses. I basically became a hermit, fearful of contact with any outside disease. My quality of life had reached the lowest point to date as my sofa and I became one, and with what little energy I had left, even receiving visitors became a chore.

After two months of this double-dose infusion, two different CT scans continued to show no change. Hence, it was recommended that I try yet another type of chemo. By this time, I was basically "punch drunk," for lack of a better term, and totally depressed about the entire process and the lack of any sign of improvement.

My local oncologist was definitely perplexed, to say the least, and admitted so, saying he had really expected some amount of regression of my cancer by this time. When I again began to question the entire process, I remembered my oncologist's comment about my will to live rather than die, and I once again decided to "take on the devil!" So, it was on to yet another chemotherapy, that being Alimta.

* * * * *

I began receiving the chemo drug Alimta in the same manner I had received the other infusions. It was recommended early on that I have a port put in, considering the large number of infusions I had had and was scheduled to receive. A chemo port is a small, implantable reservoir with a thin silicone tube that attaches to a vein. That would alleviate the need to find a healthy vein each time. It probably would have been best, but I couldn't bring myself to do it. Almost all the long-term patients had a port, and I just could not accept the idea of being a "long-term" patient.

As a side note to the chemo port discussion: I came across a very caring local group, the Gang of Seamstresses, that directly assists patients living with cancer who are personally dealing with very challenging chemo port issues. The port shirt with its shoulder seam zipper or Velcro allows access to the chest port, eliminating the need to undress.

The Gang of Seamstresses
Pat Cochran

Red Seger was going through a second go-round of cancer. I knew him since first grade. He was my friend. I wanted to do something to cheer him on. I had seen these port shirts online. They were $35 apiece. Nope. I decided I would figure it out. Three shirts from the thrift store later, they were in the mail. He wore them to his chemo treatments at The James. The nurses went crazy over them.

So, made a few more. Then a few more. And a few more. By this time the sewing group was involved. I knew they would be vital in tweaking the process, and they did not disappoint. Between all of us, we had probably close to 200 years of sewing experience. We figured it out.

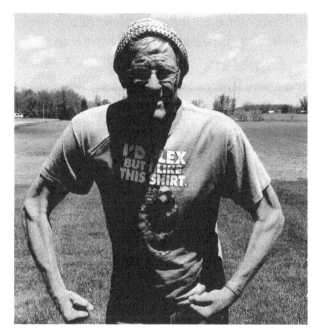

RED WEARING HIS GANG OF SEAMSTRESSES SHIRT

When Red rang the bell, the nurses said they were happy for him but sad for themselves because there wouldn't be any more shirts.

We had the thought that "duh! There are people right here who could use these shirts! "And so, the search for free shirts began with a load of about 400 soccer tees from the Beavercreek soccer group! Then donations came. More shirts. More finessing. More sewists. The need has not stopped. We send all over the United States and into Canada.

We have partnered with Turning Up the Heat on Cancer who advocates for us and helps with distribution. We are so grateful for their guidance. Without them, we might still be trying to get the world's attention.

We have gone from 3 shirts to 8500 over 3 years. Red guides from heaven these days. I bring all of this to light now because today is the anniversary of Red's death.

I thought it was time to tell the story. Red is wearing my favorite of the first three shirts made for him.

Call it a small world. As I was putting the finishing touches to my book with reference/permission requests, I had a very pleasant surprise. When checking for approval to use Red's picture, it was brought to my attention that Red was from my hometown! This, in turn, led to a very warm, nostalgic trip back in time with Red's extraordinary, strong wife, Debra. Cancer can be so very cruel to surviving loved ones.

Although a regular in the infusion room, long-term acceptance just was not in my vocabulary. For me, the infusion room, which could also include the cancer waiting room, was the most depressing place in the world. Looking around both rooms and seeing the misery and hopelessness in the patients' eyes brought tears to mine.

The steroids necessary to prevent allergic reactions before and after the infusion of Alimta added to all the other side effects that continued tearing my body down. The treatment and resulting misery that came with the infusions seemed to have no end in sight. But end, it did. After three months of pure hell, the CT scans again showed no improvement whatsoever. My oncologist shared with moist eyes that he was sorry he had not been of more help. Out of options, and after extensive research, he was going to send me to one of the best oncologists he knew. I appreciated his honesty and sincerity; I was "whipped" and didn't know how much more my body could take

Chapter 4
More of the Nasty Stuff

"Today we fight. Tomorrow, we fight.
The day after, we fight. And if this disease
plans on whipping us, it better bring a lunch,
'cause it's gonna have a long day doing it."
—Jim Beaver, Life's That Way

* * * * * * * *

It is now 2008. It has been one year since I started my treatments, and I honestly was much worse than when I had started. In reality, the year I had spent on chemotherapy regimens seemingly had done nothing but tear my body apart from the inside out. It was evident to me that I needed something else, or I would indeed die of this cancer within two years, as predicted on day one.

The doctor I was now referred to was the one most responsible for the cure of Lance Armstrong's cancer. So, it was west on I-70 to Indianapolis IUPUI Hospital and, hopefully, a new and more positive attack on my cancer.

Sadly, my bubble burst practically before the engine in my Oldsmobile could cool in the parking lot. After reviewing my files in my first meeting with the doctor, he agreed with what I had heard from previous doctors; there was no known cure for my lung cancer, no "silver bullet," if you will. I knew this deep inside, but I was looking for any little ray of hope. When I pressed that I had read that Lance had cancer in his lungs, the doctor concurred and continued that Lance also had cancer in his brain and testicles. He then noted that just because it was in the lung did not make it lung cancer. Rather, Lance had testicular cancer that had spread to his lungs and they were able to find a cure for testicular cancer. I guess I had known that, but I was hoping he might have something new for me.

He continued with the "bubble bursting" when he shared that all the chemo I had pumped into my veins the past year had likely been a waste of time!! That one shook me to the core. "Nothing, you're telling me, did any good at all?" I mumbled. He just lowered and shook his head. He did say that just as testicular cancer was incurable at one time, it was now his goal to help find a cure for lung cancer—another flicker of hope. Although my knowledge of cancer research was limited, by this time, I knew that in reality, the speed of cancer research was equal to the pace of a snail.

On a more positive note, he shared that, although the previous scans did not show any detectable remission, it did show that my cancer was slow growing. He wondered out loud about the slow growth, it was a very long shot, but there was a remote possibility that cancer had not spread to my lymph nodes as previously thought. If, by a very slim chance, the lymph nodes were swollen due to infection and not cancer, that could open up other viable options. Grasping for any little glimmer of hope, I shared I was all in for a biopsy to be sure it was indeed lung cancer causing the swelling in my lymph nodes.

The doctor pulled some strings and arranged to have a biopsy of the lymph nodes done on my next scheduled visit. I held on to the slimmest of hopes as I entered the hospital. The procedure did not take long. Literally still groggy from the anesthetic, I saw the blurry outline of the surgeon standing over me and heard another "Grim Reaper" saying, "It's cancer." The ghostly figure then quietly vanished in my anesthetic fog. After a few minutes, I came around enough to get dressed and went to where my wife was waiting. I asked if she had talked to anyone; her reply was, "No, have you?" My response was a bit hesitant, for I knew what I had just heard, but due to my groggy state, I wasn't sure if it was the surgeon or if it had been a dream! Hearing nothing else, we assumed it was indeed the "ghostly doctor of death," and I had heard him correctly. The aftermath of the procedure seemed a bit bizarre. Two words from a blurry figure while coming out of anesthesia. I was disappointed not only with the result but also with the insensitive method of informing me. The road of cancer was proving not only to be a bumpy one but also a very cruel and insensitive one at times.

Upon hearing the biopsy results, the doctor shared that our options were limited but suggested we give Tarceva another try. That was not what I wanted to hear. His rationale reinforced previous opinions: Tarceva was the only drug with any real positive effect on my lung cancer to date. I shared that Tarceva had worked me over pretty good the last time. He understood but felt it was my only viable option and possibly helped stabilize my cancer. He followed that with a recommendation to cut the dosage I had previously taken in hopes that the side effects would be tolerable.

Our ride home was a quiet one; my last thought walking into the doctor's office that day was that I would continue the use of chemotherapy. I had learned over the past year not to get my hopes up, but I honestly was hoping for something besides chemo. Anything but that damn poison! Nevertheless, I respected the doctor's opinion. He seemed on top of what was happening in the field of cancer and genuinely concerned about my situation.

The following two months on Tarceva continued to be very tough on my body as well as my mental health. The rash returned with a vengeance, while my dehydration and diarrhea caused tremendous fatigue. I was miserable, unable to do much of anything. My quality of life was at zero; I could not see any possible improvement as long as I continued on the drug.

* * * * *

On my return trip to Indianapolis, I was a wreck both physically and mentally. After the CT scan showed no noticeable change, I shared with the doctor that the Tarceva was tearing me up; the only way I could remain on the drug would be at a lower dose. He agreed and recommended a very low dose of Tarceva, hoping it would be tolerable and at the same time keep the cancer in check.

During this visit, the doctor and I discussed the possibility of a more potent pain medicine. I had been using some over-the-counter pain medicine, but it didn't seem very effective lately. The doctor did not know if the increased pain was attributed to my cancer or the large amount of chemo I had been taking. Regardless of the cause, he felt there was no reason for me to be dealing with such pain.

Now for a new, and I must say, very dark time in my cancer chemotherapy treatment, I had no experience with OxyContin, so the dire warning the pharmacist gave me as she dispensed the drug took me back a bit. As she completed the prescription, I jokingly asked about drinking a beer with the drug. She stopped, put her pen down, and in no uncertain terms, informed me OxyContin was not a drug to take lightly. And she put an exclamation mark on her comments by telling me I was not to let anyone know I was taking the drug, not even family. "People kill for this drug" was her closing comment. Although I did not realize it at the time, I would come to regret taking such a strong pain medicine.

Three more months would pass that included three additional visits to Indianapolis, along with CT scans to evaluate the status of my cancer. The last visit and scan showed no positive change and actual signs of a slight progression in my cancer.

We decided I should have a PET/CT scan for a baseline and then begin Sutent. We were now officially grasping for straws! The drug was initially developed for kidney cancer with some success, so we figured it was worth a shot. But our gun was nearly out of bullets.

I went home with hardly a glimmer of hope, fully expecting the continued misery of nausea, dehydration, diarrhea, and fatigue. A terrible way of life and something I was not willing to accept. Time crawled by, and I was not at all surprised by my miserable existence. I tried to remain as active as possible, but my body was taking a beating, and I was not able to replenish it fast enough.

*****

Another year rolled by, and I must say, not a day was without a challenge. When I returned to Indianapolis to take another PET/CT scan, it did not show any positive change. To our dismay, it again showed a slight increase in my cancer. Another doctor without any answers, stated, "I'm sorry but there is nothing more I can do at this time." He followed up by recommending that I should quit beating myself up and suspend any more chemo. Saddened but relieved at the same time, I agreed since I didn't think I or my body could take much more.

I thanked the doctor, for I genuinely believed he had made every effort possible. I asked if he would keep me abreast of any new happenings within the field of lung cancer and he assured me he would. As I slowly turned to walk out, I had one last question, "How long do I have?" Without much hesitation and moist eyes, he said that I probably would not see Christmas. Again, a quiet ride home. The silence was deafening, our minds trying to comprehend what we had just heard and calculating a short eight months until Christmas.

So it was back home to my local oncologist to discuss what had transpired in Indianapolis and where I would go next. Needless to say, I was depressed; another doctor sent me home with little or no hope.

But my local doctor was not one to give up. If he was, he certainly didn't show it. He, too, impressed by the slowness of my cancer growth, wanted to look at the slimmest of possibilities by suggesting that we take a closer look at my thyroid. Could there be the slightest chance that I had thyroid cancer, a treatable form of cancer? Anything was worth a try by this time, so he scheduled a blood test and a thyroid scan. This was beyond grasping for straws, but I thought, what the hell did I have to lose?

The cancer continued without remission and the pain had become more severe, hence the need for increased pain medication. Frighteningly, with this came an alteration in my personality that included a sensation I had never experienced before. Among other fears, I had developed a severe form of claustrophobia, which I had begun noticing when having scans performed in Indianapolis.

The straightforward thyroid scan turned out to be anything but simple. On my drive for the scan, I shared with my wife the inexplicable anxiety I was having about the procedure. Like previous times in Indianapolis, I knew it was ridiculous, but I couldn't help myself, scared that I had no idea why or how to control my emotions. This fear was something very new to me because I had always managed my emotions fairly well. The increased doses of pain medication (OxyContin) affected much more than my pain and in ways I had never imagined. So severe had my claustrophobic reaction become that the simple design of the thyroid scan machine put me into a severe panic attack. The design, which was in no way a tunnel-like enclosure but rather a machine open on all sides and requiring only a close pass over my body, should have been relaxing. Feeling ridiculous that I would have any claustrophobic reaction, yet being terrified showed the extent of my drug-induced fear—just another of the many side effects of this cancer journey that I had never expected. Fortunately, I got through the scan with an understanding technician and my wife. All the hassle and apprehension over the scan appeared to be for naught, as thyroid cancer was ruled out.

* * * * *

Others knocked on my door throughout my two years of conferring with the many doctors, experts, and specialists. One friend shared her success with acupuncture and an address for the doctor. Again, I was grasping for anything and figured, why not if acupuncture could help alleviate some of my pain? To be honest, the initial visit with the acupuncturist did seem to give me some relief, but the pain soon resumed and the herbs he concocted I literally couldn't get past my nose even when my wife tried to hide them in applesauce! I'm not sure if it was cancer or the chemotherapies, but my taste buds had really taken a beating. Food no longer had the same taste, if any taste at all. A metallic taste seemingly permeated everything I ate. Hence my appetite became non-existent and with this lower food intake came the "snowball effect:" loss of weight, less energy, and fatigue.

During the entire cancer process, I spent a great deal of time reading various medical articles and researching on the Internet. As I had shared previously, I knew I had to be my own advocate if I were ever to find an answer for my cancer. And that is exactly what I continued to do: books, journals, newspapers, TV, and most importantly, the Internet became the center of my universe. It had been recommended early on by the doctors, when asked about cancer research, to use the Internet but be selective in what sources I researched.

Due to physical fatigue, I found myself doing a great deal of reading and Internet searches, often late into the early morning hours, since sleep was very elusive at times. On one such occasion, I ran across an article in the newspaper detailing a new and successful form of radiation. This new laser radiation had the ability to pinpoint cancer and, for lack of a better word, "zap" the cancer. Previous discussions with doctors always brought an explanation that the cancer was too widespread (stage IV). Besides, radiation would probably do more harm to delicate lung tissue than help.

I was to the point of such frustration with the lack of success that I was looking for anything. My pain had increased, and I thought any reduction of cancer, particularly if it could be pinpointed, would be of benefit. I arranged a meeting with the laser doctor, but to my disappointment, he didn't want any part of my challenge after viewing my scans.

Back again with my local oncologist, he recommended yet another chemo, Gemzar. Approved as a first-line chemotherapy for lung cancer, I had bypassed it for reasons unknown to me, but without any other options, I reluctantly agreed.

Oh, what a mistake! The drug literally shook me to the bone.

Chills, fever, and nausea all hit me with an intensity I had never before experienced. What turned out to be my last trip to the infusion room. I was sitting in the chair with the Gemzar dripping into my arm when I suddenly became very, very warm. I looked at a fellow patient and asked if she felt uncomfortably warm. Looking up from her *Country Living* magazine, her smile turned into a look of horror followed by a room-rattling scream of, "Oh, my god!!"

As the nurse came running in, I felt my face and found it burning up. She immediately called for the doctor, who quickly shut off the drip and took the needle out, followed by an injection to reverse and stop the reaction. Compounding my misery, my scheduled two hours of infusion turned into three, so I could be monitored until the allergic reaction subsided. It was obvious, no more infusion for me that day, and to be honest, I had made up my mind then and there it would be the last infusion for me, forever!!

* * * * *

It had been over two years, five different chemotherapies, and two targeted therapies (some twice), and I was no closer to a cure or better quality of life than I had when I started.

I was dying, and it was not a comfortable death, if indeed such a thing exists!

As I struggled with this terrible debilitating disease, the pain was continuous. Both doctors, believing my life was nearing the end, had prescribed some very strong medicine to help me deal with the pain. Coming to the realization that I needed help with pain management, I took a trip to the Cleveland Clinic to consult a palliative care specialist. The very caring specialist discussed my pain and what I had taken previously and recommended what pain medication would be best for me. We also discussed the severe side effects I had and continued to experience. It was at this time the possibility of radiation being used to alleviate some of the pain was discussed. The doctor agreed to arrange a consultation with a radiologist to discuss that possibility.

On my return visit, I first met with the assistant radiologist and explained my hope to use laser radiation to remove some of my cancer to help alleviate my pain. I was pleased when he said he understood where I was coming from and thought it was something they could address. He had looked at my scans and even briefly described a procedure he thought could be beneficial.

Finally, someone is willing to try something besides pumping all that chemo into my body. For the first time in two years, I found myself with a glimmer of hope. After some time (I assume a talk with his assistant), the head radiologist came in and smashed any glimmer of hope, a complete reversal of what I had just heard. It took me off guard as I wondered how such completely different opinions could come from a specialist and his assistant. He basically stated what I had heard before, my cancer was too widespread and there was too much risk of damage to the lung. My argument for a simple reduction of cancer to help alleviate pain went nowhere. He countered that I shouldn't be experiencing any lung pain since the lungs had no nerve endings, hence no pain.

I couldn't believe what I was hearing. I thought, "No Pain?" He needed to be walking around with my lungs and feel the pain I felt when I coughed, sneezed, or even took a deep breath, then tell me there was no pain. Although I had not spoken, my body language gave me away, and he knew I was not happy with his response. He ended the conference with a promise that he would take my request to a hospital board of review and would be in contact. In other words, this meeting was over: "Don't call me; I'll call you."

Later, talking with other oncologists, I asked why I had such pain when there were no nerve endings in the lungs. The explanation was simple: the type of lung cancer I had was not a large mass. Rather, while I had a couple of nodes of one to two centimeters, the vast amount of my cancer was granular or sand size. When I had the opportunity to view CT scans of my lungs, I honestly had trouble actually seeing the cancer, for both lungs looked to me and my untrained eye as nothing but a smoky cloud. That, I was informed, was cancer. Trying to understand the specific cause of such pain, I asked the doctor if he could put it in layman's terms. He said the best way to explain it would be a comparison to pleurisy and the pain that accompanied it.

Now, I could not recall ever having pleurisy; people tell me if I had, I would remember, for it was excruciating. In my situation, a large amount of cancerous granular-sized nodules were near the lining of my lungs, affecting my nerve endings. The doctor also used terms such as splinters and glass shards to explain those granular-size nodules and how they might feel near the lining of the lungs. This explained the painful sensation I had each time I coughed or cleared my throat when the pain would literally bring me to my knees.

If my memory is correct, the Cleveland Radiation radiologist (I had been told he was a member of the review board to do the review) called and, as expected, stated the board had rejected my request. My mental and physical health was in a very fragile state, and I'm afraid my response was a bit gruff at best.

*****

It was June 2009, two years and two months since I was first di-agnosed with stage IV lung cancer, the maximum time doctors had given me to survive. These two years had been nothing short of horrendous; my body was ravaged. The five different chemother-apies, two targeted therapies, and the accompanying side effects had brought me to the lowest point in my life. Short walks outside became an all-out effort. Taking a shower was taxing. The sofa continued to be my haven, and reading became my one escape from reality.

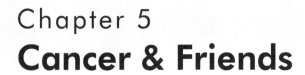

Chapter 5
Cancer & Friends

"When you go through deep waters,
I will be with you."
—Isaiah 43:2

* * * * * * * *

Fortunately, friends and family members have been very caring and supportive regarding my cancer, asking what they could do for me and letting them know when I was feeling good enough to have visitors. As I thought about my family and friends and their offers of assistance, I remembered back to before I had cancer and how I reacted to others with cancer. I was not exactly proud of myself. While I was "around" for my father, father-in-law, uncles, and best friend doing anything they asked, I'm afraid I simply had gone through the motions. I was so uncomfortable with cancer that I didn't want anything to do with it, didn't want to know anything about their cancer, nothing. Now I realized I was simply scared of cancer.

I can remember all so clearly my cousin Keith, who was like a brother, being diagnosed with esophageal cancer. As we talked and he shared his cancer journey and very difficult struggle, I listened, not because I wanted to, but because I knew he wanted me to. I look back now and think what a "wimp" I was; sorry, I did not go beyond my fear/ hesitancy and spend more quality time.

Now I find myself on the inside looking out. I am the one with cancer watching my friends, neighbors, and family struggle with the uncomfortable feeling of what to say, how to say it. I now understand and can fully appreciate the kind and thoughtful actions directed and shown to me, however insignificant they might have seemed.

When asked what to do for an individual living with cancer, I believe the best answer is to do something! Anything is better than nothing. When not sure, give them a phone call and be prepared to leave an upbeat message, for often the patient has a great deal on their plate and is just not ready for a call.

If you (or the patient) are not ready for the personal connection and are at a total loss of what to do, sending cards with notes can be an excellent idea.

Throughout my years of living with cancer, conferring with the many doctors, experts, and specialists, others were knocking on my door, a steady stream of very sincere and well-meaning individuals sharing their many unconventional ideas and methods of treatments. Well-meaning as they were, I had to smile at some of the remedies: goat's milk, a maple syrup concoction, unpasteurized milk, and herbs of all sorts were just a few of the many they shared. Some I even tried, like the maple syrup concoction, while sounding interesting, I soon found to be totally repulsive.

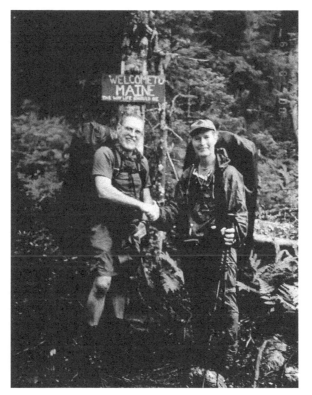

KEITH AND I ENTERING MAINE

✶✶✶✶✶

Following are a few acts of kindness that I can remember with a smile. Hopefully, the acts of kindness will help in knowing what to say and do, equally as important, what not to say or do for the person living with cancer.

- The friend who knocked on my front porch door one morning with a St. Christopher medal saying she got it in Rome, Italy, and it had been blessed by the Pope.

- The visit by a very caring former student, a clergy member. He stopped for a visit sharing faith along with some fun memories of his school days and his interaction with me as his principal.

- The good friend who stopped by our home in the country and mowed my lawn while I was gone for my two-hour infusion.

- The afternoon my wife and I came home from a very taxing day of scans and doctor visits to see one of my best friends and his wife weeding the flower beds and cleaning around our pond.

- I can't begin to express my gratitude for all the prayer chains I was included in throughout the community.

- The neighbor driving his John Deere tractor up to our home in a blowing snowstorm to clear snow out of our driveway, knowing that we would be traveling out of town for a doctor's visit early the following morning.

- The gift of sharing books with my brother-in-law and close friend as they sent me books they had read and later followed up with a phone call or visit to discuss them. They may never know how that small act of kindness to get my mind off my cancer was so helpful.

- The 90-year-old neighbor who stopped by with a gallon of goat's milk confident that it would "cure" my cancer—sharing his story of years back as a young lad. When a team of horses broke loose from the hitch pulling him across 10 acres of ground before he got them stopped after breaking numerous vertebrae in his neck, the doctors said he would never walk again. After a year's diet of "only" goat's milk, he was up again the following spring planting behind the same team of horses, much stronger and wiser! Sadly the old gentleman passed away at the ripe old age of 99, taking with him a wealth of information that will sadly be lost to the ages. I believe there is an old African proverb that goes something like this, "When an elder dies, a library burns to the ground."

– The brother-in-law who rode his bike 30 miles to my house to ask my advice about long-distance bike riding, knowing biking had been one of my passions before my cancer diagnosis. That made my day! Sadly, he was taken from us way too soon.

– My wife's cousin, realizing the numerous trips we were taking for hospital and doctor visits, was thoughtful enough to send gas cards.

– My neighbor's front porch, where he and I sat for hours and watched the wildlife meander by while we solved the world's problems.

– An act of kindness that I know had to take a great deal of time and thought were the personal notes of encouragement sent weekly by one individual during the first two years of my cancer journey.

A snack always seems to bring a smile. A particular memory was my father-in-law's request for pork rinds following a rather uncomfortable day at the infusion center. Everyone in the car discouraged his snack choice, but his ear-to-ear smile of satisfaction is a lasting memory. With that said, checking to make sure the food item would be permitted is always advisable. That also applies to gifts of plants and flowers, which are sometimes inappropriate. You certainly do not want to be responsible for any complications.

If possible, get your friend living with cancer out of the house. Take a walk or a short ride in the country if mobility is problematic. I'll never forget my high school buddy who cleaned and polished his antique lime green Ford Fairlane and drove to my house to take me out for a spin to pick up the well-known local "Maid-Rite" sandwich, reminiscent of the old days.

*****

Favorite Visit: He arrived one morning, unannounced, on a two-wheeled cart pulled by a little Shetland pony. I wasn't having a particularly good day when he and his pony came clip-clopping down the Ol' Grey Pike into our lane. A high school classmate I had not seen for a while, a friend but not a really close friend, so I was very surprised. Did I say I was not having a particularly good day? Well, by the time he had jumped back on the cart and was clip-clopping back down the road, my spirits were lifted from all our reminiscing/laughing and I was looking forward to his next visit. As he left, I had a smile on my face and a tear of appreciation on my cheek, so happy he had come. Five years later, I visited this friend on his sofa at his home just months before he succumbed to cancer.

I came to cherish friendships found in the strangest of places that often evolved into everlasting friendships. Some were fleeting encounters leaving just as much of a memory as a longtime friendship. In a smelly, cramped infusion room filled with what I called "lounge chairs of misery" sat a lady who happened to have been from my hometown. She would always stand out in my mind. Beginning only as a casual acquaintance within the confines of the infusion room, we developed a pleasant friendship in a relatively brief time. When sitting side by side with poison being pumped through a needle into your vein, you really get to know that person in a very unique and personal way. I found it much easier talking with someone going through the same misery and could relate. As we sat and talked, there were days when no one escaped our wrath: doctors, relatives; we were giving them all hell. Sadly, the day came much too soon when the chemo just became too much; and she left this world for hopefully a more genteel afterlife.

While having an enjoyable visit is excellent medicine for an individual living with cancer, there is something to be said for calling ahead. One morning I had a well-meaning relative knocking on my door with her young daughter in tow. Now, who does not want to see their young niece, right? Sadly, at that very moment, I was lying in my front room with a lap full of vomit. I apologize for being so graphic, but obviously, I was not ready for visitors; a call would have been best for all involved.

*****

Along with being sure to call before a patient visit, I have a few suggestions of what "not" to do:

- It typically does not benefit anyone to share negative stories about other individuals living with cancer to make them feel better.

- Don't assume that the patient can't hear you, even if they seem to be asleep.

- I have found it is not advisable to offer medical advice or your opinions on things like diet, vitamins, and herbal therapies unless asked.

- It is essential that the patient's decisions about how their cancer will be treated is theirs and needs to be respected, even if you disagree.

- Avoid saying, "I know what you're going through."

- Be very careful not to ask the caregiver questions about the patient while the individual is within hearing distance.

- Quiet time can be good; you do not need to be talking the entire visit. Just being there is fine.

*****

Last but not least, don't forget the caregiver; they can always use a break. Often called respite care, giving the caregiver a little time out of the house can be beneficial. This relief from the around-the-clock responsibility can come from family members, friends, and charity organizations that may be available.

A quick call to offer assistance in picking up groceries or, better yet, an offer to stop by for an hour or so visit that allows the care-giver a chance to do some shopping or just "chill out" is always welcome.

Another consideration for the caregiver is in the form of finan-cial assistance. A full-time caregiver obviously cannot work outside the house, so knowing there are possible avenues for assistance is beneficial. One is the National Family Caregiver Support Program which often provides financial support for those caring for relatives aged 60 or older.

Not sure how to explain this, but when helping the caregiver, it's imperative to listen—an example. In a doctor's office waiting room, I overheard a dad explaining how worried he was about his wife to his two adult daughters. Every example of his wife's behav-ior that concerned him was met with the daughters' disagreement. They were not listening! The moist eyes of the father were painful to witness.

When in doubt of how to help a caregiver, offer to do anything: help with some chores, offer to pick up the kids if applicable, cook, clean house (I know, ugh!), pick up medicines. I believe you get the message.

Concerning caregivers, encourage a support group or grief counseling, a safe place to share their feelings.

*****

Final thoughts: I have seen the ugly face of cancer from every angle in family and friends, children and adults, young and old. I have seen it in their eyes and tears; I have looked in the mirror only to see cancer looking back at me. I know how mean and nasty cancer can be for all my family, friends,

and neighbors. I judge no one on their behavior toward an individual with cancer.

Now that I have shared my thoughts and ideas about supporting a person living with cancer, please know that you may find many more ideas and suggestions from organizations such as the American Cancer Society and the National Cancer Benefits Center.

Chapter 6
Hope at Last!

"Cancer may have started the fight, but I will finish it."
—gotCancer.org

* * * * * * * *

Then it happened. The date and event that saved my life will forever be etched in my mind. On June 9, 2009, ABC World News with Charles Gibson aired a brief segment on a new drug for lung cancer under study in Boston.

An attractive, healthy-looking young lady by the name of Linnea Olson stated, "I have adenocarcinoma non-small cell lung cancer, and it is now melting away." Specifically, the words "melting away" exploded out of the TV at me. Springing from the sofa, I exclaimed, "That's me, adenocarcinoma non-small cell lung cancer, stage IV." I couldn't believe I had just heard someone use the very words describing my specific lung cancer, let alone say it was "melting away." I had been lying on the sofa watching the news but not really listening and just caught those final few words. I looked at my wife and asked if she had heard the comment that I thought I had heard. She also had been "half-listening" and only heard the final few words of the segment. We did not have a system to record programs then, so I went sprinting (let's call it a hurried walk) to the computer to see if I could download the ABC news program. Nothing about the cancer segment popped up; evidently, the program segment was not yet available on their website.

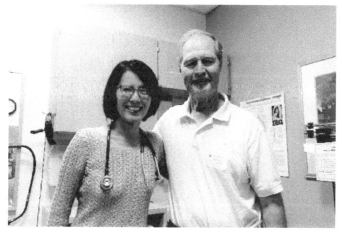

DR. ALICE SHAW AND I AT AN MGH VISIT

It was a day or so before I sat down at my computer and read the entire news segment that had aired. In my reading, I was able to locate the doctor's name, Dr. Alice Shaw, and the hospital, Massachusetts General Hospital (MGH), currently conducting the study. (MGH is now known as Mass General Brigham) Information about the patient Linnea, who had been featured, included she was a relatively young individual and most important to me, she had been a non-smoker.

I had to keep pinching and reminding myself that there had been many promises in the past regarding cancer without any real benefit to my cancer. Nevertheless, I whipped off an email to the oncologist in Indianapolis and a doctor in Cleveland who I knew would contact my oncologist at the clinic. I immediately heard back from the doctor in Indianapolis, and he shared he had actually been at the conference where the study results were featured and the news clip was filmed. If I had the opportunity to get into the clinical trial, he certainly would recommend it. The response from the oncologist in Cleveland was not as positive. He reiterated his belief that I had exhausted all treatments available to me. By now, I had had my fill of the extremely pessimistic oncologist and was not about to allow his negativity to deter me!

Hearing such positive results from the news segment and the doctor's support in Indianapolis, I felt it certainly warranted the email I sent to Dr. Shaw at MGH in Massachusetts. To say I was pleasantly surprised when I received an immediate reply to my email would be an understatement. Her request for a phone number and a personal conference was beyond my expectation. I eagerly e-mailed my phone number and promptly received a personal call from Dr. Shaw, in which she gave me a very detailed description of the study. The fundamental aspect of the study was the development of a targeted drug aimed at a specific type of lung cancer. It was explained that I would have to qualify for the study by having a sample of my cancer tumor DNA tested. My tumor samples would be checked for a specific DNA translocation that they found would respond well to a targeted drug Pfizer had developed. When asked to explain in layman's terms how the drug worked, Dr. Shaw described that the specific translocation acted as a light switch stuck in the on position. She continued by saying the targeted drug works to turn off the switch, therefore reducing cancer cell production. This was an excellent explanation of the complex nature of the targeted drug and its ability to control a specific cancer.

Dr. Shaw also stated that only a small percentage (3 to 5 percent) of lung cancers had the specific DNA makeup in their cancer cells that had been receptive to the targeted drug. I would need to get a sample of my lung cancer biopsy to MGH then they would perform the DNA testing. She asked if I was interested and, if so, suggested that I get the sample to them and make a visit to MGH for a consultation. The advanced consultation at MGH would help speed up the process if I was a match and qualified to participate in the clinical trial. She asked how I felt about a trip to Boston, and without hesitation, I exclaimed, "I'll be there tomorrow!" We both laughed, but I did reiterate that I was "all in" for the possibility of qualifying for the trial. I said I would immediately begin sending her my current reports, have the biopsy samples sent, and make arrangements for travel to Boston.

I was elated with the thought of possibly being part of this cutting-edge study on targeted drugs. Although I began faxing information to Dr. Shaw the next day, the challenges of finding usable biopsy tissue from the hospitals took a lot more time than I had anticipated.

*****

During this time, my wife and I arranged to drive to California via the Glacier and Crater Lake National Parks. As my health continued its decline and no longer on any weekly chemo treatments, I began to give serious thought that this may well be my last opportunity for any extensive travel. Along with seeing the National Parks, I was also looking forward to a visit with my youngest son and his family in Redding, California. Naturally, I couldn't help but wonder that, due to my failing health condition and the travel distance between us, this could be my last opportunity to see and spend time with them.

I had loved traveling by auto, but my cancer caused a great deal of nausea, fatigue, and pain, turning the drive into a real challenge. This trip was compounded by the anxiety of obtaining a good biopsy sample to send for a DNA analyst. Apparently, the hospital in Indianapolis had lost my most recent biopsy, so we had to rely on the original sample taken in Cleveland to be large enough for analysis. Fortunately, Dr. Shaw worked with us while on the road. We eventually were able to get all the proper release forms needed by Cleveland. We completed them using faxes from Crater Lake with the help of both my daughter-in-law in California and Dr. Shaw in Boston.

The final episode in this drama was the challenges in the return trip home. We had purchased a newer automobile for the large amount of driving we anticipated would be required between MGH in Boston and home in Ohio, so I arranged to drive and transfer my older car to my son in California. We arrived in California with my older automobile via the National Parks and had scheduled to fly home. Incredibly by this time, my claustrophobia and panic attacks from the pain medicine had become so severe that I absolutely could not fly on a plane. I was a mess. I awoke in a cold sweat at three in the morning, scared to death at the thought of flying in an airplane with no chance of escape. And this was not even the day of the flight. The thought of being confined in that tiny aluminum capsule was overwhelming and had me pacing the floor of my hotel room. My dilemma was eventually solved with my son's assistance, who found us a rental car so we could drive the two thousand-plus miles home. I was not going to let anything stop me from getting to Boston!

Finally, all the paperwork was completed, and the biopsy sample was sent to Boston. About two weeks later, I received word that the sample would be enough to complete the analysis, and my wife and I finally arrived at MGH to meet with Dr. Shaw. What a lady! I was not only impressed with her vast knowledge of lung cancer and the targeted drug possibilities but her enthusiasm and positive attitude were contagious. The visit went well, and now it was just a matter of waiting for results from the DNA testing to see if I was ALK (Anaplastic Lymphoma Kinase) positive, thus making me eligible for the clinical trial. I knew the percentage was low, something like only 4 percent of individuals living with lung cancer had the ALK mutation, but Dr. Shaw shared she had a good feeling about my chances. Needless to say, the waiting was pressure-packed. I would find waiting and cancer to be joined at the hip throughout my cancer journey!

Chapter 7
Targeted Drugs & Clinical Trials

*"Be strong, be fearless, be beautiful.
And believe that anything is possible when
you have the right people there to support you."*
—Misty Copeland

* * * * * * * * *

The call came ten days later. Great news! I had tested positive for ALK, but... I was not ready for any "but." There was a need to retest, something about not quite an exact match, and a requirement to verify. I had not quizzed Dr. Shaw on the reason for a retest, so the next week of waiting was terribly nerve-racking with the uncertainty. The results came with another call from Dr. Shaw, who happened to be in California for a conference. Realizing the extent of my anxiety, she took time on a Saturday to inform me everything was a go. It is impossible to express my relief when told I qualified for the study. I even detected a tone of excitement in the very professional Dr. Shaw's voice as we scheduled my appointments for the study at MGH.

With high hopes, Connie and I arrived at MGH to begin preparation for the clinical trial. We met with the Phase I team, who outlined the study procedures and administered a battery of tests to establish a baseline. All the tests were routine: physical, blood work, and CT scan, except for the required "dreaded" brain MRI. I would not qualify for the trial if cancer were found in my brain. Evidently, the drug was not very effective in penetrating the brain. Therefore, any tumors in the brain would have to be dealt with before starting the study. So, the one-day wait was another unexpected delay and caused more anxiety. I learned early on that living with anxiety is the norm for all individuals living with lung cancer. As I signed the consent form, the team reviewed possible side effects: fatigue, nausea, diarrhea, and vomiting, in addition to visual blurring and acid reflux. Of note, there was a specific concern about the liver function and the need to be monitored closely. The team also discussed the limited results to date of the trial from current patients using the study drug:

60% of current trial participants were considered "partial responsive," meaning a 30% or greater shrinkage of the baseline tumor.

20% of current trial participants were considered "stable disease," meaning a minor shrinkage or stabilization of the baseline tumor.

17% of current trial participants were "non-responsive." I didn't ask what happened to the other 3%!

August 12, 2009, day 1 of the Clinical Trial, marked the beginning of a new phase of my life's battle against lung cancer. It had been over two years since my devastating original diagnosis of stage IV lung cancer, two years of "pure hell" that had diminished my body and soul to a mere shadow of existence. Now I had been thrown one final lifeline. It was all I had, and I was determined to do everything in my power to hang on.

*****

Nine a.m. I was directed to a hospital room in MGH where my phase 1 team of Sarah, Jose, and Marguerite were stationed with pills, clipboards, and anxious looks. Also, in the tiny, anxiety-filled room were Dr. Alice Shaw and her assistant, a fellow, Dr. Bhatt. With the watch in hand, the team dispensed my three pills totaling 250 milligrams, referred to as PF-02341066 (later known as Crizotinib). They were given to me to take with water on an empty stomach. The three pills, two times a day at 12-hour intervals, would be my allotted dosage throughout the study. Then it was watch and wait, with the team recording on their different clipboards a variety of observations. After about an hour, feeling like a mouse in a cage, I began to get a little restless just sitting on the bed and asked if it would be OK to get up and walk around a little. With a reassuring yes from the team, I got up and immediately became a little woozy. Feeling sick to my stomach, I made a "beeline" to the bathroom, where I promptly vomited into the toilet. A bit embarrassed and fearful that I had vomited up my first dose and even possibly ruined my continuation in the study. I sheepishly walked back into the room. Seeing the concern in my eyes, the team told me not to worry; enough time had elapsed for the drug to have entered my system.

Now here is where it became extremely interesting. I find myself hesitant to share this part of the story due to the amazing happenings. While talking with the team, I noticed a somewhat puzzled/concerned look on my wife's face after I had re-entered the room, but I was too involved in what was happening to talk with her at the time. After the commotion settled, Connie approached me and whispered, "Are you OK?" I said, "Yea, I guess so." She continued to look at me with that look of "You sure?" and I asked a bit irritably, "What is it?" Then it struck me; she didn't need to say more. I had not exhibited any pain at all! We both stood open-mouthed in disbelief. For the past two years, the pain in my chest had constantly increased to the point, particularly whenever I coughed or sneezed, that it would literally bring me to my knees. Despite the strong dose of OxyContin I was currently taking, I found I also needed a breakthrough pain pill at least four times a day, especially for moments like this when I coughed, choked, etc. And here I was, standing in the room without any pain after bending over the toilet and heaving my guts out! I could not believe it and, as I have told others many times, I never really expected them to believe me. And if it had not happened to me personally. I would not have believed it myself.

Later, I shared this response with Dr. Shaw expecting a surprised expression, but she simply responded that the drug seemed to affect individuals in different ways and usually very quickly. The rest of the day involved close monitoring and four additional blood workups. After my second dose, I was released in the early evening and would return the following morning for more blood work and observation to ensure I was doing OK.

The next day went well; I was doing "normal," whatever that meant, and my blood work looked good. So I was released, study drug in hand, to go home with instructions to call Dr. Shaw if I began feeling poorly or had any concerns. I was also scheduled to return in two weeks for more blood work and observations; this would be the routine for the next eight weeks, with the "all-important" first trial CT scan at the end of that time period.

During the next eight weeks, our every-other-week, 1700-mile round-trip drive to Boston was very relaxing and uneventful. Especially gratifying to me was the lack of pain, hence no need for any breakthrough pills and a decreased dosage of pain medication. To monitor my condition, we arranged with my local doctor's office to fax blood work to Dr. Shaw at MGH the week I did not travel to Boston.

On my next trip to MGH, Dr. Shaw showed me the CT scan taken on the first day of the trial as the baseline and compared it with a CT scan taken after my initial diagnosis in 2007. The baseline showed quite an advance in my cancer when compared to the early CT.

I had asked Dr. Shaw at the onset of the trial if there would be any signs that would give me an indication of a positive response to the targeted drug. I vividly remember her comment, "You'll know before we will." I wasn't sure exactly what she meant at the time, but with the disappearance of that deep pain I had felt for so long, years! I wondered to myself if that was what she was talking about. But it was far too early to be so optimistic, and I fought the urge to be overconfident even though I felt so much better.

*****

After a relaxed week at home, I began a reversal in my condition, which started with severe back and stomach pain. I reverted back to the pain breakthrough pill while experiencing a great deal of stomach pain and vomiting. Thinking it was possible side effects from the drug, I tried to endure the pain; but it got so severe I finally relented and had Connie drive me to the local ER. By the time I entered the hospital, I was doubled over in pain. The ER nurse had me admitted and seen by a doctor who immediately ordered blood work and an X-ray. He returned, saying I had blood in my urine. My heart sank. I told him I had lung cancer and was on a clinical trial, then waited to hear the worst. The cancer comment raised his eyebrows a bit; then he said not to panic and that he needed time to check some other test.

Although it seemed like an eternity, I'm sure it was fairly quick when he came in and said, "I have good news and bad news." That was not what I wanted to hear! My mind had been racing with the many devastating scenarios, and I told him in no uncertain terms not to mess with me and give it to me straight! He saw my frustration and quickly shared that the bad news was I had kidney stones, and the good news was I had already passed them. I don't believe there was ever a happier man on this earth to hear that he had kidney stones than me!

With the taxing and exhausting experience at the ER over, I was ready to move on. The next six weeks encompassed blood work at my local hospital and, every two weeks, a visit to MGH for additional blood work and consultations with Dr. Shaw and the Phase 1 team. I continued to experience fatigue, nausea, and a new sensation, flashes of light at various times throughout the day. One dynamic that continued to change throughout this period was my reduction of pain medicine, and by the end of the eight weeks, I was down to 10 milligrams of OxyContin three times a day and no breakthrough pill. This was down from a high of 80 milligrams. Now the significant reduction of pain medicine was quickly becoming a challenge in itself. Although an obvious positive, the rapid decrease in pain medicine was having an effect on my body for which I was not at all prepared. My body began to indicate a need for OxyContin, even though the pain for which I was taking the pain medication had basically subsided. The palliative care doctor I had been working with constantly cautioned me about rapidly reducing my pain medication. But I was so happy to no longer need the medication and wanted to no longer deal with those side effects which accompany the medicine. I'm afraid I may have "pushed the envelope" a bit too fast.

Chapter 8
High Fives All Around

"You beat cancer by how you live, why you live, and in the manner in which you live."
—Stuart Scott

* * * * * * * *

The end of eight weeks found me at Chelsea Lab in Boston having my first CT scan since being on the clinical trial. The scan was a "walk in the park" compared to the terrible liquid substance required of me to drink within their one-hour time limit. The two-quart bottles of the dreadful contrast I forced down brought me very near to the delicate point of vomiting it all over their waiting room floor. I wondered to myself how I would ever be able to drink the putrid stuff for future scans.

The scan was on a Friday, and my appointment with Dr. Shaw and Dr. Bhatt would be the following week to discuss the results. Physically, I had been feeling pretty good the last few weeks leading up to the CT, but I had so many disappointments in the past concerning CT scans that I was extremely apprehensive. As I sat in the hospital room awaiting the results, the doctors wheeled the computer in with a copy of the scans; and before I could even ask, both Dr. Shaw and Dr. Bhatt were "high-fiving" each other, I immediately thought, "Man, this is surreal." Now, I had observed many different reactions by doctors throughout my time in the various hospitals, but never had I seen "high fives." Needless to say, my scans showed excellent results: a large number of small granular-size nodules were gone, and the views of both lungs were remarkably clearer than the baseline CT just eight weeks earlier. The three tumors identified on the baseline CT for measurement and the four lymph nodes along the esophagus were all significantly smaller. I was on cloud nine. I could not have been happier; for the first time since my lung cancer diagnosis, I was seeing a positive response. There had never been hope before, and now there WAS hope. I felt I could actually start making plans again. Two absolutely miserable and terrible years with seven different poisons pumped into my body had brought me to my knees; a targeted therapy was finally working. Not to be overly dramatic, but the clinical trial drug Crizotinib looked to be saving my life, at least for the time being, and I would take it each and every day!

In consultation with the doctors, we discussed the results in detail. With all the immeasurable granular size nodules eliminated, the official trial measurements did not show the total picture of a positive response. Therefore, on the official clinical trial status, I was listed as "partial responsive." But as stated, the doctors were as elated as I was, and now I would continue taking the targeted drug and hope for continued positive response. The other good news was that I could forgo every other week trips to MGH and begin a monthly drive to Boston, with weekly blood work and check-ups completed at home with my local oncologist and faxed to Dr. Shaw and the Phase 1 team.

* * * * *

My first visit to my local oncologist for the needed blood work and checkup is one that will be everlastingly etched in my mind. As I entered the office to check in for my appointment, my local oncologist was looking over some papers. He casually glanced up, back down, then with a snap of the neck, he looked back at me with the face of seeing a ghost. When I last left his office a year ago, my condition had deteriorated to the point that I am sure, he never expected to see me again. After a minute or two of awkward silence, his first comment was to point out how good I looked. The last time he had seen me, I was at the end of my physical limits; cancer and different chemo's had turned my relatively healthy body into a frail shadow of my previous self.

"I thought you were dead!"

He exclaimed as he entered the exam room. I smiled and shared information about the clinical trial I was involved with and the success I had to date. He was stunned, asking me for specifics of the study as he hurried out of the room to his office, where he quickly returned, lugging his enormously thick 2009 medical journal. As he rapidly fingered through the pages, constantly asking for the trial name and number, he shook his head, pointing to the few short lines in small letters highlighting the study I had described. What jumped out at him was that it was a Phase 1 study, and shared, as he shook his head in wonderment, that he would have never recommended me for a phase 1 study, even if, by the slightest of chances, he would have seen this one study out of the thousands listed. This illustrated how difficult it was for local oncologists to stay updated on the latest advancements in every cancer. It would be nice to see some form of technology to help doctors stay up to date in real-time. Yet, I could tell he was ecstatic over my success and stated with a smile as wide as the room, "You just made my day." The doctor went on to say he would be more than happy to help me with blood work, CTs, or anything that could help me in my successful battle against cancer. Shaking, no, pumping my hand as I left the room, he exclaimed, "You just added years to my life!"

* * * * *

As the days rolled by, I slowly began to gain weight and strength; fatigue became less of a factor. One of the most obvious changes for me using the targeted drug was my improved quality of life. The targeted drug was so much better than the previous chemos, which seemingly attacked any cell they touched with reckless abandon, good or bad. Another wonderful benefit was the ability to continue reducing pain medication, albeit at a slower pace, to decrease the withdrawal effects that continued to plague me.

On the fourth month of the trial, I had my regularly scheduled blood work performed early in the morning, then met with Dr. Shaw and Dr. Bhatt for my consultation/check-up. As had become standard practice, it was on to the Phase 1 team, who administered the drug, completed the paperwork necessary for the study, and supplied me with enough of the drug to last the following month until my next visit. On this particular visit, the ever-so-diligent Dr. Shaw noted that my blood work indicated a deficient phosphorus level. She provided a prescription that hopefully would help return the level to normal.

I began looking forward to the monthly visits as I could have the questions my wife and I had jotted down answered, as we developed a very close, positive, and trusting relationship with both doctors and the Phase 1 team members. Developing that close relationship was not a difficult task because the professionalism of the team was so pervasive. A prime example was Sara, the study nurse who administered and dispensed my study drug. She took over the challenging duties of a phlebotomist. I believe phlebotomists are the unheralded "angels" of the hospital world. The typical patient sitting in the waiting room probably doesn't even know their name, let alone the medical label attached to their profession. Yet, speaking as a needle-scarred patient of the cancer wars who has sat in the phlebotomy lab for literally hundreds of blood draws, I have an acute awareness and appreciation for the phlebotomists and their varied skill levels. As someone who has sat and watched as the thin silver needle slides oh so smoothly and painlessly into my vein, I quickly came to admire the skill involved in such an undertaking. Sadly, I have also sat and watched as a not-so-angel-like phlebotomist aggressively jabbed, then jabbed the needle again into my arm with the forcefulness of a farmer pitching hay, with zero success of finding a vein.

Chapter 9
Sharing the Good News

"When cancer happens,
you don't put life on hold.
You live now."
—Fabi Powell

* * * * * * * *

Dr. Shaw had contacted me before my visit and asked how I felt about sharing the positive experience I had so far on the clinical trial with others. I said sure but was somewhat surprised and a little apprehensive when she mentioned ABC World News. But I quickly got over the apprehension and was so happy with my results to date that I relished the opportunity to share the success of the drug with others, particularly due to the fact ABC World News was how I first learned of the drug and its success.

During my November visit (Lung Cancer Month), along with others involved in the trial, I was interviewed for an ABC World News with Charles Gibson segment by John McKenzie. I shared a little about my positive experience. John McKenzie was a true professional who made me feel very at ease throughout the interview. Mr. McKenzie appeared to be very knowledgeable about lung cancer and its challenges, sharing that ABC World News had a particular interest in lung cancer as it had taken the life of one of their own, Peter Jennings. Dr. Shaw later told me the hospital received calls from all over the country from individuals diagnosed with lung cancer desperate for answers and looking for hope after the ABC news segment. This response was certainly gratifying. Not only was I an active recipient of this cutting-edge breakthrough in lung cancer treatment, but I was also able to be actively involved in getting the message out to others.

Days rolled by throughout November as I continued the reduction of my pain medication to the point that, by the 29th of November, I was entirely off OxyContin and all forms of pain medication. This achievement even surprised my fine palliative care physician, Dr. Terence Gutgsell.

My second CT, since the start of the trial, was also completed; and the good news continued with more reduction of cancer nodules, thus indicating a further positive response. Another decision from the "powers to be" involved using a liquid contrast that I was required to drink before my CT scans. It was, as stated previously, some nasty stuff. I had asked that due to the number of CT scans

70

I was receiving for clinical trial purposes, could the liquid contrast required for the CT be eliminated. Anyone who has had the unfortunate occasion to drink the liquid contrast for a CT would know precisely what I am talking about, and I'm sure would side with me on this one. Much to my delight, the request was granted. Despite this change in contrast protocol, I regularly found myself challenged by some overly zealous technicians.

Another welcome decision was made before my fifth CT scan since the beginning of the trial. In April, Dr. Shaw allowed me to complete it at our local hospital and have the results mailed to her and the phase 1 team at MGH. This change allowed us to avoid a weekend layover in Boston each eight-week CT scan cycle. The fifth scan was again exceptional, indicating continued shrinkage of the tumors to a total measurement of 59%!

The progression of positive response in my tumors to date had been:

1st scan 14% response
2nd scan 30% response
3rd scan 42% response
4th scan 44% response
5th scan 59% response

* * * * *

April 1, 2010. I was really back into the swing of things, basically doing whatever I wanted to do. The only side effect that hindered my activities was the occasional bout with diarrhea. This I struggled to control through diet and anti-diarrhea capsules. The side effects of diarrhea seemed to have a snowball effect on other concerns, such as low phosphorus and general fatigue. Besides walking, swimming had become a major activity for me. Before the clinical trial, I had tried swimming with the hope of building up some strength. Still, I quickly found that breathing deeply enough to swim was no longer possible with the combination of my cancer, chemotherapy, and pain medication. But now, with the cancer reduced by over half in my lungs, the hardcore chemo and pain medication eliminated, I could breathe and swim without difficulty.

I entered the pool with a tremendous fervor and eventually accomplished my goal of swimming 100 miles over a period of several months. I could even get back on the Appalachian Trail (a trail I had thru-hiked in 2000) for a few days with a cousin, something I had previously thought would never happen again. I was ecstatic! It was difficult to put into words the elation of being so close to death, and now I was back swimming and hiking. I told myself that never again would I take for granted the simple plea-sures of life. I had a second lease on life and was going to enjoy each and every day!

Around this time, Dr. Shaw asked if I would share my story again, this time for a medical journal. She put me in touch with Dan Ferber for the Howard Hughes Medical Institute. Mr. Ferber's article in the Nov. '10 HHMI bulletin entitled "Exposing Cancer's Soft Spot" is, in my non-professional opinion, the most informa-tive article I have read to date. Giving a very detailed, clear, and concise account of the targeted drug Crizotinib, the very informed and diligent Ferber was able to fuse just enough technical terms with layman's terms to satisfy the various levels of knowledge any reader might possess.

* * * * *

My August 10, 2010, scheduled visit to MGH was somewhat of a milestone; it had been one year since I had entered the Clinical Trial. With the blood work complete, Dr. Shaw reviewed my CT scan and was encouraged that my positive response continued to look stable. There had been some questionable shadows on the previous scan. They were not present on the current scans, so there was relief that the shadows were probably inflammation and not any kind of cancer recurrence.

More good news for my wife and me, Dr. Shaw had received the approval from study coordinators to allow me to forgo my monthly visit to MGH in exchange for bi-monthly visits. Blood work would need to continue, but the monthly blood work and bi-monthly CTs could now be completed at home, with results sent to Dr. Shaw and the Phase 1 team. This certainly would be a saving in travel expenses as well as a noticeable saving in time. Feeling like I had taken so many CTs and my body had absorbed enough radiation to light a darkened room, I continued pushing Dr. Shaw for fewer CTs. That was part of the clinical trial protocol and would need approval, possibly at a later date. Although aware of my concern over the large amount of radiation, Dr. Shaw was reluctant to extend the time span between CTs for fear of missing any change in my cancer status. As she told me early on when they were very concerned about my stage IV cancer growth, "Radiation is the least of your worries." The large number of CT scans continues to be a concern and has become an ongoing issue echoed by many of my clinical trial cohorts.

Chapter 10
Quality of Life Never So Good

*"Life is short and the world is wide,
the sooner you start exploring it, the better."*
—Simon Raven

* * * * * * * *

As the days and weeks flew by, my check-ups and blood work remained stable and uneventful, which was good news for everyone. Of some concern was the occasional leg pain and swelling, usually after prolonged sitting, a concern expressed by many on Crizotinib. Dr. Shaw recommended I try some pressure socks and make every effort to get up and walk whenever possible during long drives and flights. With improved health, I was more physically active, and we traveled a great deal more both in the states and abroad. Hopefully, the socks and walking, when possible, would help reduce leg pain and swelling. I had always loved to travel, so when my health improved, I immediately began to look at side trip possibilities (Lake Placid, NY, and Acadia National Park in Maine) which could be interwoven with our regularly scheduled trips to MGH. We even worked in an occasional afternoon walk along the Appalachian Trail as we crossed the trail for our numerous appointments in Boston.

As time passed, my thru-hike of the Appalachian Trail in the year 2000 seemed to pull on me with greater intensity. Each time we came to a crossing of the AT, the longing for the trail proved to be much stronger than before. The 2,167-mile trek from Georgia to Maine left me 30 pounds lighter, and after one hundred and fifty-three days on the trail, I was exhausted to the point that, when asked by trail enthusiasts if I ever considered hiking the trail again, I quickly replied with a "Hell no!" That being said, I regularly find the AT seeping out of me at times and occasionally bursting out of me, as had occurred on the last visit to Boston when we stopped at a rest area for a coffee. Spying a Pop-Tart, I thought, why not? When I went to pay, it was six dollars. I thought, "Wow, this coffee price is out of control!" When the clerk told me the Pop Tart was $2.89, the next words out of my mouth were straight from the trail as I exclaimed, "That's trail food, for heaven's sake!" It took me just a minute to compose myself and remember that what I used as a snack on the trail for a quarter was now a gourmet meal.

I also became very busy researching on the Internet and began arranging "bucket list" trips like cruises of the Adriatic and

Mediterranean Seas. I even talked Connie into purchasing and re-storing an old Airstream Argosy travel trailer we saw sitting along the roadside on one of our trips east. We then took off on a long-planned ten-thousand-mile cross-country adventure along the Alaskan Canadian Highway to Denali National Park.

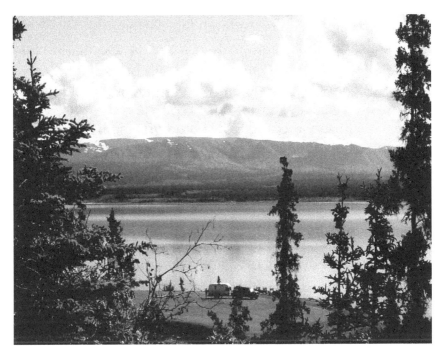

LUNCH BREAK, REST AREA ALASKA-CANADIAN HIGHWAY

* * * * *

As we entered 2011, I could not have been happier. My cancer remained stable a year and a half into the clinical trial. More im-portantly, my quality of life had been at an all-time high since my cancer diagnosis in April 2007. Dr. Shaw and the phase 1 team continued to be there for me by email or phone. A monthly check-up did not go by that I did not hear from a doctor. Even when the checkup was completed at my home hospital, Dr. Shaw or a col-league would call to follow up and answer any possible questions.

Throughout this time, I received many inquiries from individ-uals (usually prompted by one of the interviews) who either had some form of lung cancer or had a friend with cancer. And I never tired of sharing my cancer experience and positive results, giving as much information, and spending as much time as they would want. What would remain etched in my mind forever was the total hopelessness I had felt at times when it seemed like no one had an answer, and I swore to myself that I would do whatever was necessary to help anyone faced with this dilemma.

On one specific occasion, I had a cousin who had a friend who had a friend whose mother had recently been diagnosed with lung cancer and was devastated. When asked if I would talk with her, I said of course and encouraged a phone call so we could get together. The husband called and shared that they were just a few miles north of me in the next county. I invited them to our home, and within a few days, they were sitting on my sofa telling her story. Without going into great detail, the non-smoking young mother, with two children in high school, looked in excellent health and had been totally floored by the lung cancer diagnosis. Like me, the diagnosis had come out of nowhere, and she also was stage IV, with no hope. I asked the all-important question of whether or not she had had a DNA analysis of her cancer biopsy and got the usual puzzled look and response of "No." Sadly, many oncologists were not doing DNA analysis at the time, and I was not sure where she could go to complete an analysis. I typically would have suggested she have her doctor investigate the possibility, and if there was any reluctance by the doctor, to run, not walk, as fast as she could and find a doctor who would do an analysis. I could tell by the desperation on this lady's face that she needed more. I was never comfortable giving Dr. Shaw's phone number to others, but I felt the lady's pain so intensely that I went ahead and asked her to let Dr. Shaw know I had given her the number. What happened next is all that needs to be said about Dr. Shaw and her devotion to people with cancer.

The lady sitting on my sofa just four hours earlier was now on the phone, voice quivering. She had called Dr. Shaw's number as soon as she arrived home and, to her amazement, was able to talk with Dr. Shaw personally. And what brought her to tears of joy was Dr. Shaw's willingness to spend over an hour talking with her about her diagnosis, informing her of all the possibilities and options, and even recommending where to go for DNA analysis.

The next time I talked to Dr. Shaw, I apologized for not checking with her first before giving out her phone number. Sharing, I was just caught up in the lady's immediate need for help. Without any reservation, Dr. Shaw insisted that I never hesitate to direct someone her way when in need of help. As I have stated, "What a lady!"

* * * * *

Around this time, my leg pain, although not severe or debilitating, continued to bother me; although simply a common side effect in the study, Dr. Shaw thought to be on the safe side that I should get a bone scan. What a relief when the bone scan returned negative, so I continued with a calcium and phosphorus supplement.

Another one of the side effects not previously discussed but becoming more of a concern for me involved gaining weight. On monthly visits, the standard questions about how I was feeling would typically be asked, and I would share the usual challenge of diarrhea, leg pain, etc. Inevitably Dr. Shaw would ask with a sly smile, "So, how's the appetite?" This she already knew (all one had to do was look at the belly I was developing), and her smile was in anticipation of what had become my typical response of "too good." Of course, for a cancer doctor, a healthy appetite could never be "too good." As I shared my frustration with putting on weight, she shared that the complaint had become more commonplace among clinical trial patients, particularly women. Not sure if this little "tidbit" of information was to make me feel better, but it did little to alleviate my frustration with the increase around my midsection. But again, looking at the total picture, I knew full well that the alternative of lung cancer ravishing my body was not even an option. I would continue to watch my diet and try to control the additional weight with exercise, knowing the importance of eating healthy and keeping up my energy level.

Another milestone, at least for me. As I had shared previously, I was constantly lobbying Dr. Shaw about reducing the number of CTs required for the study. The approval finally came through; Dr. Shaw shared that I would now be permitted to have the CT scans every four months, even though she was hesitant about the time between scans and the possibility of not catching the cancer if it became unstable. It had been shared often with me, and I knew full well by this point that my cancer was not curable. Far from it, it could and likely would become active again. The return of Linnea's (female patient I had first seen on ABC World News) cancer further emphasized this, causing her to seek other targeted drug options. Still, I had been subjected to many high-level CTs, and I just wanted to limit the number if possible. I was hopeful that my cancer was slow-growing enough that the danger of recurring cancer would be detected.

*****

June of 2011 brought more opportunities to share my success and good fortune with a newspaper article in the Boston Globe and a second Nightly News interview.

The Boston Globe article by Carolyn Johnson, "Targeted drugs aid in cancer treatment," came as cancer specialists met in Chicago to share results of current clinical trials and other findings. Dr. Shaw was one of the presenters who shared the results of the Clinical Trial Crizotinib and the amazing response to date. Ms. Johnson neatly tied these results in with my success and how I had learned about the targeted drug on a TV news program. While the clinical trial participants were relatively small in number, the positive responses of patients like me certainly were encouraging for the future of all targeted drugs being developed by Pfizer and other pharmaceutical companies.

The second national news interview was with Scott Pelley of CBS, his first night on the air, and I found it very intriguing how the whole thing fell into place. Less than two hours before the CBS Evening News was to air, the satellite truck sent to record and send

my interview back to New York for the segment was still maneu-
vering around in my Ohio barnyard trying to locate the satellite.
I thought there was no way it would happen, but it did happen;
just before air time, I was sitting in a lawn chair in my backyard
talking to Dr. Jonathan LaPook, the CBS news correspondent. With
Dr. LaPook asking questions via phone, I could share my story with
him and Mr. Pelley back in New York for the Evening News broadcast, along with individuals worldwide. What a wonderful feeling
to be able to share the news about a drug that literally saved my
life with the many individuals living with lung cancer who, like me,
were previously told to simply "go home and make arrangements.
There is nothing else that can be done."

The next four months before my scheduled CT scan was relatively uneventful, with blood work and doctor visits pretty routine.
The only challenge was an occasionally lost fax between my local
hospital and MGH, a minor problem when looking at the total
picture but very frustrating nonetheless.

My August visit to MGH was the first since I had gone to four-
month intervals between CT scans, and I was a little anxious to
see if there was any notable change in my cancer. Sadly, Dr. Shaw
was not there, nor was Marguerite, the nurse practitioner. Nothing against the doctor who filled in for Dr. Shaw, but she simply
was not as knowledgeable about the clinical trial and seemed to
ask me more questions than I did of her. What I did take away
from the meeting during my visit was the recent FDA approval of
the trial drug Crizotinib, now marketed as Xalkori. Of course, this
approval would obviously affect me directly, and I had many questions, but none I assumed needed to be addressed immediately.

* * * * *

December brought another CT scan, and my anxiety about
a four-month interval instead of two months was more than anticipated. But the scan was stable, and Dr. Shaw continued to be
delighted with the scans and my ability to do just about any activity
I desired. This was illustrated by a 130-mile bike ride I took with

a couple of friends in the fall. We rode from Pittsburgh, PA, to Cumberland, MD, on The Great Allegheny Passage, a converted rails-to-trails bikeway. We had scheduled this bike ride around one of my Boston visits. Connie and I met my bicycling friends in Cumberland, where they parked their car then rode with my wife and me to Pittsburgh. We began our bike ride east to Cumberland, and Connie continued home to Ohio.

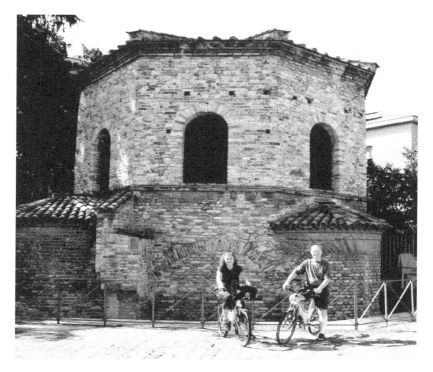

BIKE TOUR OF RAVENNA, ITALY

Another adventure quickly followed the bike ride, although a bit less physically demanding: a cruise out of Venice, Italy, on the Adriatic Sea with a lot of walking on the various shore excursions. The ability to bike long miles and travel extensively was something I never thought I would ever be able to do again, so I was determined to take full advantage of my so-called "second lease on life."

I awoke one morning thinking how lucky I've been since my diagnosis five years ago to have had the opportunity to travel the world with "relative" ease. I say that with caution thinking about the many challenges of needing a restroom at the most inopportune time, such as the sudden urgent need when boarding a boat for a one-hour ride through the canals of Venice.

During my December visit with Dr. Shaw and the CT scan review, we also discussed in detail the FDA approval of the trial drug Crizotinib (Xalkori) and its implications for me. Basically Pfizer, the pharmaceutical company that developed the new targeted drug, agreed to keep all current clinical trial participants in the study for as long as the individual patient wished to do so. Of course, that was a no-brainer for those patients who did not have a health insurance plan that covered the cost of the drug, which was predicted to be around ten thousand a month. I was in a little different position. I had checked with my health insurance and found relief that they currently covered the new FDA-approved drug Xalkori at a tier three copay level.

We also traveled a round-trip distance of 1,700 miles on each visit to MGH in Boston, resulting in high travel costs. A point of interest: Connie and I sat down once and figured since the beginning of the clinical trial, we had traveled to MGH in Boston 27 times for a total of 47,600 miles. So, I had to weigh the travel cost while considering other factors, such as no guarantee that my insurance would not change their policy at some time and the fact that I would be switching to Medicare in the near future.

Also in the equation was the realization that this drug was not a cure, and the likelihood that, at some point in time, my lung cancer would mutate around this drug was a real possibility shared by all involved. Finally, I had to consider that Dr. Shaw was the one person I trusted with my life, and I knew I wanted her in "my corner," regardless of how many miles I would need to travel. Dr. Shaw quickly assured me that she would remain my oncologist for as long as I wanted her, so it was my decision as to whether I would stay in the trial or opt out. After weighing all the pros and cons of staying or leaving the study, I decided to continue for the time being, realizing I could remove myself from the study at any time.

The new year brought continued good health (at least as good as one could expect living with lung cancer), another cruise, this time to the Caribbean, and an opportunity for me to fulfill a long-time desire of a visit to a Mayan archaeological site in Central America. I had the good fortune in years past to visit the ancient ruins of the Romans and Greeks in many countries throughout Europe but had not traveled to the relatively close Mayan Empire. So, when I came across a January bargain cruise to the Caribbean, we took advantage of it.

Again, once I was diagnosed with a terminal disease and had somewhat of a reprieve, I was not letting any "grass grow under my feet!" The only drawback to a cruise of this type is that it puts me in close proximity to a large number of people on a relatively enclosed venue, that being the cruise ship. Of course, there was also the element of traveling to Third World countries and all the challenges that came with travel in that part of the world. Hence, returning home, I found myself fighting a suspected sinus infection, if not something worse. An antibiotic was prescribed, and my subsequent blood work at MGH indicated that my white blood cell count was normal.

Chapter 11
It Never Ends — A Bump in the Road

*"You can be a victim of cancer, or a survivor of cancer.
It's a mindset."*
—Dave Pelzer

****

In April 2012, I returned to MGH for another CT scan, which showed my cancer continued to be stable. It had been five years to the month (an enormous milestone in lung cancer) since I had been diagnosed. Truly amazing! I was beating the odds. The "six months to two years" prediction by previous oncologists had come and gone. I was still walking this earth and loving life thanks totally to Dr. Shaw, the phase 1 team, Pfizer, and the targeted drug Crizotinib.

While reviewing my regular blood work, Dr. Shaw suggested I may want to see an endocrinologist because my testosterone was normal, but the binding was low. After a more detailed and extensive test by the endocrinologist, the results were not at all what I had wanted to hear. My PSA was 9, way above where it should be, and now red flags indicated the possibility of prostate cancer. My first thought was, "You've got to be kidding me!" What is the chance of a person having two cancers at once?

I was directed to yet another doctor, a urologist, who would hopefully give me some answers. The high PSA number and the knowledge that other family members had prostate cancer certainly indicated a strong possibility that I could have it. When I shared my current battle with lung cancer, an eyebrow of the doctor raised with an expected "Oh no." And instead of a specific recommendation which I was looking for, I got the, "well, you can get a biopsy, or take some pills in the hope that it's just an infection, or do nothing." The "do nothing" came out very matter-of-factly, and I got the distinct feeling he was thinking, "Hell, the lung cancer is going to kill this guy anyway and probably sooner than any testicular cancer."

When I voiced my thoughts, the silence and hesitant nod of his head readily reaffirmed my belief. I really didn't know what to do, so when I asked him what he would do, a shrug of the shoulders and an "It's your decision" was not the response I had hoped to hear. Noting there didn't seem to be any urgency and not relishing the thought of a biopsy on my posterior, I elected for the antibiotic and another blood test in a month. From within came the "sixth sense" of a person living with lung cancer that told me I was just putting off the inevitable. A month passed, and to my surprise, a significant drop in the PSA number to 4 was shown on the blood work. Although a good sign, it simply meant that if it was growing, it was a slow-growing cancer; again, the same options were given. Not wanting the knife to my posterior, I elected to go another month on pills looking for "God" knows what, a miracle, I guess. No miracle, the numbers increased. I decided to bite the bullet and go with a biopsy. My only regret was not doing it right away.

Wow. That was not fun! I was told a prostate biopsy would not be much, a quick in-office procedure that would go quickly and uneventfully. I soon learned that what I had been told was putting it at the lower end (no pun intended) of the anxiety scale. My first indication of anything being amiss was the amiable and pleasant little man with all his photography gear as I entered the room.

Having never met the doctor who was to perform the biopsy, I was not sure if this little fellow was my doctor. So not wanting to be rude, I sat back for a few minutes and carried on a very uncomfortable bit of chit-chat. Finally, my curiosity overcame my ability to carry on this charade of relaxed conversation, and I asked with as much politeness as I had within me who exactly he was. The jovial fellow smiled and answered, "No doctor. I'm just your friendly little photographer," as he went about untangling wires, programming his software, and whatever else was needed to come away with a beautifully clear picture of the inner workings of my prostate.

With everything up and running, the doc finally entered the room and did his thing. There was a casual conversation between the doc and me, with me asking most of the questions. His comments centered around, "We're almost done. How are you doing?" Finished with the procedure, the doc and his friendly smiling photographer stood, arms out, awaiting me to collapse flat on my face. It never happened. I couldn't wait to get out of that rectal torture chamber; no further assistance would be needed!

A very brief meeting to discuss the biopsy results came a few weeks later with a report of what I had dreaded but was fully prepared to hear. When I asked my options, he glossed over them rapidly and was very non-committal about radiation, surgery, or just doing nothing. Again, I could see in his eyes that he figured I was going to die of lung cancer, so what the hell.

*****

Not wasting any more time, I was out of his office and on the phone with Dr. Shaw. She suggested two options, have treatment at home or travel to Boston. She would arrange a consultation with three knowledgeable colleagues: a surgeon, a radiation oncologist, and an oncologist, to discuss my options. That was a no-brainer; I jumped at the opportunity to get all the options in one setting and be able to ask questions of all three.

April 22, 2013. I was sitting in an MGH conference room with three specialists, very pleased they had all reviewed my biopsy and came in with recommendations. All spoke, but to my surprise, the oncologist deferred to the surgeon, who did not recommend surgery. Instead, he gave reasons why he thought radiation would be my best option, then referred me to the radiation oncologist. The radiation oncologist covered the radiation options if that was what I elected to do. All three doctors were in total agreement.

I could not have been more pleased with the input and my decision was quick. I elected the IMRT (Intensity-Modulated Radiation Treatment). Dr. E would be heading up the radiation, and although some newer and less invasive radiation treatments, such as proton, were available, he felt the best option for me would be IMRT. I shared that the typical nine-week schedule was a challenge considering our travel distance and the need to find lodging. He suggested the possibility of five and one-half weeks at a higher dose which had been successful for patients with my health and scores, so I jumped at it. The suggestion of lodging at the Hope Lodge cemented the decision. Another advantage of MGH was the close proximity of Dr. Shaw; I was the first patient Dr. Shaw had on Crizotinib who would be having radiation treatment simultaneously.

Located within seven miles of MGH, the Hope Lodge was established for any adult cancer patient living fifty miles or more outside Boston. Truly a great facility. Dr. E's office began the paperwork, and with some luck on our side, a room was available. Our final concern with being away from home for such an extended time was the matter of home maintenance. Patients often overlook this issue due to the overload of things they must consider. Fortunately, our friends watched our home while we were gone and occasionally volunteered to mow grass and do general yard work.

*****

One of the negatives of being part of a clinical trial is the many rules and regulations, officially referred to as a protocol. A specific rule of my Crizotinib Clinical Trial was no other cancer treatment while on trial. Fortunately, Crizotinib had been FDA-approved. I could now access the drug with a prescription under the brand name Xalkori. My decision to leave the clinical trial was somewhat mixed. Without sounding too sentimental, it was a little like losing a close friend. I would still be taking Crizotinib under the new name Xalkori; I would no longer be meeting with the Phase I clinical trial team I had worked with for the past three and one-half years. Connie and I would miss the team members' encouragement and support as we had come to know them personally. Of course, Dr. Shaw would continue to be my primary oncologist.

My daily radiation treatments that were to last for five and a half weeks were painless and lasted only ten minutes. Although only ten minutes, the machines had a tendency to break down. That's not what a patient, required to lie under a machine shooting a million "zaps" of whatever into their body, wants to hear.

*****

The most significant benefit of the short radiation treatment time was just that, short time. The doctors told me slight fatigue was all I should expect as a side effect. So, feeling good, Connie and I started to stretch our legs by seeing Boston up close and personal with bike rides, walking the Emerald Necklace Parks, John Quincy Adams Homestead, JFK Boyhood home, and of course, Fenway Park, to name a few.

Our most adventurous weekend was a trip to Mt. Washington, New Hampshire—one of my favorite stops along the Appalachian Trail during my thru-hike in 2000. I had always hoped to share the breathtaking summit of Mt. Washington with my wife. Share it, we did. After a nice leisurely Clog Train ride to the top of Mt. Washington, we decided to hike down the AT trail to Lake of the Clouds Hut for an evening dinner, overnight stay, and breakfast. Early the following day, instead of the Clog Train, I suggested we hike the rest of the way down, or should I say slide down! Connie was a real trooper in agreeing to hike down, but I, the experienced thru-hiker, should have known better. It was not pretty, considering the steepness of the ice-covered terrain. We made it down, scratched, bruised, and ready for a nice, warm, bone-soaking bath.

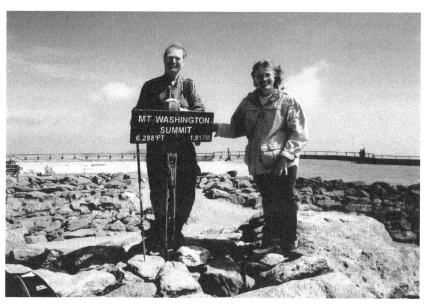

WINDY SPRING SUMMIT OF MT. WASHINGTON NH

* * * * *

I "rang the bell" at my final radiation treatment hurrah, and while the Hope Lodge had been comfortable, we were anxious to get home. Sad again to be leaving newfound friends; there is a special bond naturally present when two or more individuals living with cancer meet. I walked away with one especially memorable friendship that began the first day we met. "Old #43," and I hit it off right away. He was a member of the 1963 Championship Chicago Bears. We could sit and lie to each other for hours. Besides the naturally competitive nature between a Chicago Bear and a lifelong Green Bay Packer fan, yours truly, we both connected with stories of our past coaching days.

Chapter 12
Did I Say it Never Ends?

*"You never know how strong you are
until being strong is the only choice you have."*
—Cayla Mills

* * * * * * * *

All patients diagnosed with terminal cancer and fighting the ultimate battle have two constant fears, like a millstone around your neck lingering in the far reaches of your mind: Will it come back? Will it spread?

I came across this article early one morning while browsing through Facebook, posted by an ALK patient. I thought it "hit the mark!"

4/12/2021

Imagine you're going about your day, minding your own business, when someone sneaks up behind you. You feel something press up against the back of your head, as someone whispers in your ear. "Sssshhhhh.... don't turn around. Just listen. I am holding a gun against the back of your head. I'm going to keep it there. I'm going to follow you around like this every day, for the rest of your life."

"I'm going to press a bit harder, every so often, just to remind you I'm here, but you need to try your best to ignore me, to move on with your life. Act like I'm not here, but don't you ever forget... one day I may just pull the trigger... or maybe I won't. Isn't this going to be a fun game?" This is what it is like to be diagnosed with cancer. Any STAGE of cancer. Any KIND of cancer. Remission does not change the constant fear. It never truly goes away. It's always in the back of your mind. Please, if you have a loved one who has ever been diagnosed with cancer, remember this. They may never talk about it or they may talk about it often. Listen to them. They aren't asking you to make it better. They want you to sit with them in their fear... their sadness... their anger... just for the moment. That's it.

Don't try to talk them out of how they are feeling. That doesn't help. It will only make them feel like what they are going through is being minimized. Don't remind them of all the good things they still have in their life. They know. They are grateful. But some days they are more aware of that gun

pressing into the back of their head and they need to talk about it. Offer them an ear.
Written by Sherry McAllister

Going on three years of stable CT scans indicating no progression, my confidence had increased. Maybe, just maybe, we were on to something more permanent?

Life had been good since my return from Boston after the radiation treatments. Family reunions, National Park trips, oldest son Bruce's Change of Command ceremony, and bike rides had replaced long drives to Boston for CT scans.

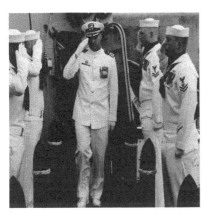

BRUCE, CHANGE OF COMMAND

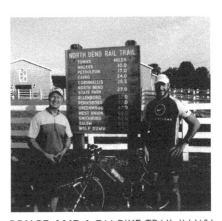

BRUCE AND I ON BIKE TRAIL IN WV

On a late October visit to Boston, a scheduled meeting with the radiation doctor showed a clean report and was followed by a clean CT scan from Dr. Shaw. During my visit with Dr. Shaw, I mentioned being a bit more unsteady than usual, at which point she suggested a brain MRI may be warranted. I had been on Xalkori for four-plus years, and knowing what I know now (that Xalkori was not as effective in protecting the brain), I probably should have had a brain MRI sooner.

It was late in the day when Dr. Shaw found the only available MRI machine in Chelsea, which happened to be off MGH's main campus, so we hopped in the car and drove across town. What I thought would be a routine check-in, get your scan, check-out soon became very frustrating. While filling out the extensive MRI form, I checked a box sharing that a sliver of metal had been removed from my eye years ago. The wheels of the scanning world at Chelsea stopped! MRI technicians practically came sprinting out of their tiny lead-clad rooms, telling me I had to have my eye checked for metal, and even though I had had at least one MRI at MGH since the removal of the metal, they weren't buying it. To make matters worse, all the X-ray machines in-house were in use; my only alternative would be to get an X-ray in one of their other buildings. It was late, and we had made arrangements to watch our grandchildren in Long Island, two hundred and fifty miles away, a five-hour drive. I had had enough! So, we left.

* * * * *

After an enjoyable weekend with the grandkids and with Long Island in our rear-view mirror, I was relaxing on my sofa in our living room ten hours later. The MRI was completed a day later at the local hospital, where Connie and I enjoyed a cup of coffee while awaiting the results, which would then be FedExed to Dr. Shaw at MGH. Our relaxing coffee break was interrupted by the ring of my cell phone. It was the MRI radiologist, "Have you left the building?" That doesn't sound good, I thought. "You need to see your doctor before you leave." Now I knew it wasn't good! Fortunately, we had an appointment with the local oncologist, so I hitched up my big boy pants and prepared myself for some bad news.

There was no waiting. As we entered the office, we were shown directly to an exam room; the doctor came in within minutes. The look on his face told the story. "It's not good," he shared, as he began to read my report that stated I had several small brain Mets and one rather large one. I found myself surprisingly calm; I guess I had expected this, and although very disappointed, I was in no way shocked or flabbergasted.

On the other hand, I was a bit perplexed by the oncologist's anxious talk and speed of action. Immediately after sharing my report, he was making phone calls and arrangements for me to see specific specialists for treatments. My mind was still somewhat abuzz with the terrible news that I had brain Mets, that my lung cancer had entered my brain! I knew it was possible, and I knew it would more than likely happen, but I just was not quite ready for someone to tell me it had. Words were coming out of the doctor's mouth that I did not want to hear and was not prepared to hear.

My hand finally went up like a traffic cop on the corner with a big "whoa," when I heard the words "Whole Brain Radiation!"

Meaning no offense to my local oncologist, but I knew how important it was for me to say no, or in my case, "whoa," when I was uncomfortable with the direction the local oncologist was going. (If I had gone along with the standard treatment recommendation, I would have had my "brain fried" with whole-brain radiation! There may be a time for whole brain radiation, but I believe that should be an alternative best held off for as long as possible.)

The oncologist was a partner to my regular local oncologist, so he didn't know me or my individual situation very well. The "whoa" had gotten his attention. As he looked up from where he was busy scribbling out a prescription for steroids and the names of different specialists, I calmly explained we needed to make one phone call: Dr. Alice Shaw at Massachusetts General Hospital. A bit of puzzlement appeared about how we would call Dr. Shaw until my wife handed him a phone number and calmly shared, "You're a doctor. I'm sure you can get through." Five minutes later, he was back in the exam room with a confident smile, tearing up the steroid prescription he had written and saying with a somewhat surprised voice, "I got right through! There will be a different plan. Dr. Shaw will be calling you."

My abrupt "whoa" resulted from six years of living with lung cancer and research on the hazards of whole brain radiation, including a wonderful team in Boston whom I relied on for their expertise.

Later that day, Dr. Shaw called with a plan of action. On my next trip to Boston, I would meet a neurosurgeon for a scheduled pre-op conference followed the next day with surgery. I would be in the hospital for two to four days with an expected recovery time of two weeks. Surgery would be to remove my largest tumor with the remaining three small Mets eliminated with laser surgery, SRS (Stereotactic Radiosurgery).

*****

So, it was back to Boston. During the pre-op conference, we discussed the following; 90% tumor removal and SRS laser surgery to complete tumor removal. Vision at risk due to the location was mentioned, as well as stopping Xalkori for two days.

The surgery went well and was shorter than expected, with me up and walking the halls in no time. My initial talk with the surgeon after the surgery started with the obvious question. "Did you get it all?" He followed with "NO." My heart sank. He said, "You don't want me scraping around in your brain." He finished with, "Radiation will be used to finish the job."

Dr. Shaw stopped in and laid out the drug options available to me that would better penetrate the blood-brain barrier to prevent the recurrence of brain Mets. Options presented to me were: Chugai(Alectinib), LDK(Ceritinib), AP26113(Brigatinib), PF06463922(Lorlatinib). All four options were clinical trial drugs; three were second-generation ALK inhibitors and the fourth was a third-generation inhibitor. After reviewing the pros and cons of each option, Dr. Shaw suggested that I take some time and give the options some thought; we would make a decision at a later date.

The next day Dr. Shih, my radiation oncologist, came in to explain what would happen next in my treatment plan. She explained SRS and how the focal radiation treatment would work on the remains of the primary tumor, using five to ten low-dose treatments. The three small brain Mets would be a single treatment for each. These treatments would start one month after my surgery if all went well during the healing process. So hopefully, I would have my treatments completed by Christmas.

I had two weeks of recovery time before I could go home, and a great deal of the time was used on trips back and forth to MGH for checkups and prep work. Thank goodness we were able to arrange lodging at the Beacon House, which was conveniently within walking distance of MGH. Dare I say quite the walk up Beacon Hill! Arranged through MGH, accommodations at the Beacon House are offered to patients of MGH at a very reasonable discount.

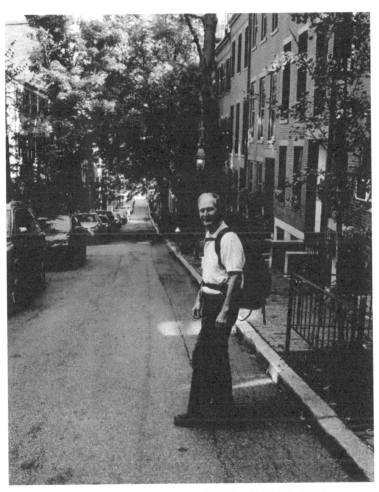

BEACON HILL ON THE WAY DOWN TO MGH

The prep work involved creating a head device, similar to a football helmet, that would be used during my radiation treatments. A personally constructed device involved me meeting with a technician who took my head measurements, then built a perfect-fitting helmet that locked down to the table, ensuring no movement. I was glad they took so much time to ensure the fit was exact, for the precise treatment to be administered by the laser beam to my brain was crucial. The final days of my recovery included a wonderful surprise visit from my daughter and grandkids, followed by the removal of my stitches and a very welcomed exit for home.

One of the extraordinary friendships I developed on my cancer journey was Royce Burt, an outstanding violin luthier. He went out of his way to give me a little cheer and diversion after my brain surgery by sending my revoiced violin (fiddle) to me in Boston. This valuable diversion from the reality of cancer cannot be understated, although not sure if the other patients in the adjoining rooms shared my enthusiasm.

* * * * *

On Dec. 9, 2013, I was back in Boston after a two-week recovery from my brain surgery to prepare for SRS radiation treatments to clean up the area around my surgically removed tumor and the three small brain Mets. Before beginning the radiation, we met with Dr. Shaw to determine which of the second-generation ALK inhibitors that were known to penetrate the blood-brain barrier I would be going to next. While the four inhibitors had benefits and drawbacks, we selected the Alectinib (Chugai) Clinical Trial with Dr. Shaw's guidance and input.

The one major drawback to the clinical trial was a very demanding protocol that would require a great deal of travel time. To our relief, we found the Alectinib Trial was open at the James Cancer Center in Columbus, Ohio. That looked to be a no-brainer when comparing the 1700-mile round trip to Boston and the Columbus 200-mile round trip. Dr. Shaw understood our travel challenge and was supportive, so we called the James Cancer Center for information on the Alectinib Trial and set up a Jan. 6th appointment to complete the screening process and begin the study. In talking with the clinical trial coordinator at the James Cancer Center, there was a great deal of information required, and we assured them we would make every effort to get it all collected and sent to them on time. Which we accomplished after a great deal of time and effort.

Dr. Shih started my radiation treatment the day after we arrived. With just two weeks of rest after surgery, I was still a little weak and had shared with both doctors that my energy level was pretty low. They concurred that was expected and attributed it to the surgery and the steroids I had been taking to keep the swelling down in my brain. The radiation sessions went well, but my energy level continued to decline to the point that I was sleeping a lot more, and climbing stairs became more of a challenge.

On Dec. 23, I was ringing the cancer radiation bell again, this time equally happy to be yanking on the rope but a lot more exhausted. The combination of surgery, travel, and more radiation treatments was beginning to take a real toll on my body. We had made arrangements to visit my daughter and family on Long Island as we traveled home from Boston, which we typically did, but probably not the best decision after all I had undergone.

But visit we did; not only did we visit the kids on Long Island, but we also took a trip into the city with them to see the Christmas Tree at Rockefeller Center and the famed Rockettes. While I enjoyed the city and loved being with the grandkids, I was one worn-out grandpa as we headed home to the Buckeye State and some much-needed rest. Being a grandpa, is there anything better?

I often think of my seven grandchildren and can't help but think how fortunate I am. Not often do you find a stage IV person living with lung cancer talk about how fortunate he is, but there I was saying just that. I simply remember back ten years to my diagnosis of stage IV lung cancer and predicted life expectancy of two years. Four of my seven grandchildren have been born since then and have blessed our family. Who could ask for more?

* * * * *

The following day at home, I found myself still totally exhausted. The doctors had assured me that, considering the surgery and radiation I had gone through, the extreme fatigue I was experiencing could be expected. But the intense headaches were unexpected; combined with my apparent sinus infection, I dragged myself from bed to sofa.

A call to the local doctor and a bit of pleading on the part of my wife got me squeezed in for an appointment. We filled the doctor in about my latest bout with surgery and radiation, and

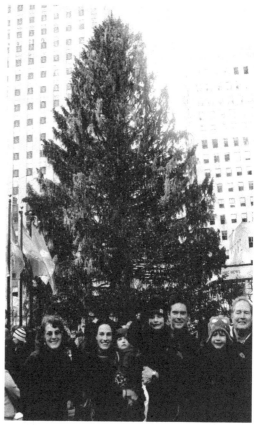

DAUGHTER, ELIZABETH & FAMILY

after a quick check-up, he concluded I indeed did have a severe sinus infection. With that, he gave me a three-day dose of an antibiotic called a Z-Pack with the instructions to get right back to his office if I did not show improvement.

Three days later, I was back in the doctor's office feeling just as exhausted and stuffed up, it not more so, than when I was last in his office. The doctor again looked me over. He could tell I was one wiped-out individual and prescribed another round of antibiotics and a pocket full of antihistamines and decongestants. He prefaced it with a warning that since we were right at the holiday season, it was imperative that if I did not begin to improve immediately, do not wait around and get medical help immediately.

* * * * *

"Ringing in the 2014 New Year" could not have been more adventurous. An hour after midnight on New Year's Day, I crawled off my sofa and staggered to the stairs for my bedroom. The next thing I knew, I was face down with my chin bouncing down each step like a rubber ball, landing in a fetal position at the bottom of the stairs.

By this time, my wife was downstairs shaking me and saying we needed to get to the hospital now! All evening I had been vacillating about going to the hospital; I now realized I had no choice, very aware I had been wrong in putting an earlier hospital trip off. As I began to dress, Connie mentioned an ambulance; it was probably the right call, but I didn't want the "fuss" and asked her to get the car.

I don't remember much about the forty-minute ride to Upper Valley Medical Center, but the arrival was memorable. As I rolled myself out of the passenger door in what seemed to be slow motion, I told Connie to park the car. I would be OK. Lightheaded and weak in the knees, I slowly staggered to the emergency room entrance. If it were not for the quick-acting receptionist and her "Rosie the Riveter"- like arm strength, I definitely would have done a "face plant" right there in the reception area.

After being helped to a wheelchair, my extremely low oxygen level hastened a variety of tests; respiratory distress was the term used as they wheeled me into the ER. Not sure when, but rather early on, I mentioned that I had Stage IV Lung Cancer and noted the doctor's glance at me with a nod of acknowledgment. A quick X-ray showed evidence my sinus infection had evolved into pneumonia in both lungs, resulting in a state that the doctor shared in a somewhat non-medical term as a "mess."

As my breathing moderated and I began to stabilize, the ER doctor explained all the treatments she had ordered and asked if there were any other concerns as she was about to go off duty. I was feeling much better and wondered aloud how soon I could leave. She smiled, saying I was not going anywhere just yet. She had decided that with everything I had gone through in the past month, surgery, radiation, pneumonia, and lung cancer, it might be best to do a quick chest CT scan.

Oh, thank the Lord for the ER doctor and CT scan. To our surprise, not only did I have "a mess" in my lungs, but the CT clearly identified it as a large blood clot. While not at all happy about the blood clot, I was elated it had been discovered before it caused any more damage. That changed everything; there would be no going home now. On January 1, 2014, I was being wheeled to a hospital room with a life-threatening blood clot.

Never having experienced anything like a blood clot, I didn't know what to expect. But I was totally blown out of the water when I was put on oxygen and given a blood thinner, and when I again asked about going home was totally ignored. It didn't get any better as the day progressed, and the on-call doctor, making his rounds, came in to check on me. Somewhat of a gruff fellow, he was pretty direct, which I liked, but he seemed in a big rush. (I know, aren't they all?) He got my attention when I casually asked if he was ready to release me. "Release you? Listen here; you're lucky to be alive. Over half the people with a blood clot the size of yours never walk out of the hospital." Dr. Positive continued that my release would be awhile, depending on getting my numbers right, oxygen level up, and so on; so, we were looking at a week or more. "Are you serious?" I asked. I couldn't believe what I was hearing; I just nodded, knowing nothing more I could say was going to influence him.

Rejoicing in the knowledge that Dr. Positive had left for the rest of the day. My hope of getting an early exit from the hospital was tempered by the nurses keeping an eye on my numbers, specifically my oxygen. I was exhausted. It had been a long day and, in all likelihood, would be a long night. Throughout the night, the oxygen tube in my nose was continually falling out, sounding an alarm, making for a very sleepless night. I casually asked the nurse how long I would have to be on oxygen, whereby she matter-of-factly said with a smirk and all the seriousness of a Himalayan Monk, "The rest of your life." That is what I fell back to sleep hearing. To say I was bummed out would certainly be an understatement; I just had a major setback, a life-threatening setback. I had just been through major brain surgery and radiation and was getting ready for another targeted drug that would possibly extend my life, and now this. So as I drifted off to sleep on New Year's Day 2014, it didn't seem like it could get much worse.

*****

Ah, but the sun came up the next day with rays of hope. The first "ray of hope" came after our communication with Dr. Shaw in Boston, updating her on all that had transpired the previous day. We were able to send copies of all my numbers and a copy of the CT scan and drugs that had been administered. She was great, looking over all the info and getting back immediately. In particular, she requested the change from the blood thinner Coumadin to Lovenox to be aligned with Clinical Trial protocol.

The second "ray of hope" was another pulmonologist making her rounds. I had already conferred with Dr. Shaw and had a list of needs and questions. I told the doctor immediately that I was living with stage IV lung cancer and had an oncologist at MGH in Boston whom I hoped she would consult. "Of course I will," she replied with a bright smile, "Let's see what we can work out." That was music to my ears. Some hope and positive feedback are what I was looking for and, quite honestly, needed at the time.

The day continued from good to great as I learned from the doctor that the biggest reason I had to stay in the hospital was my oxygen level and the monitoring of my blood thinner. Now that I had changed the type of blood thinner, that was no longer an issue; so, all we had to deal with was my oxygen, and if I could get home health oxygen delivered to my home that day, I was free to go.

I couldn't believe my ears; I went from a week or so in the hospital to home in a day if my oxygen arrived on time. They informed me that I would need to continue on oxygen until I could maintain a level of 93%, which could be weeks or even months.

While I was surprised at the length of time they were saying, I was very weak and knew that the extra oxygen supply was vital in my present condition.

As the day progressed and my oxygen level stabilized, it became obvious that I would be going home that day, so the scramble for an oxygen company/supply began. Weak but one happy man, I remarkably left the hospital, albeit in tow of clanking cylinders of oxygen and disapproving head shakes.

One not-so-small detail not discussed but was shared with me just before leaving the hospital concerned my need for a blood thinner on a continuous basis. What really set me back on my heels was the explanation of exactly what they meant by "on a continuous basis," that being for life!

Since I had a blood clot and, incidentally, blood clots and lung cancer go hand in hand, I was now required to have a daily injection (blood thinner.) Being the wimp I was, I really was not up to sticking a sharp little object in my tender-like belly anytime, let alone daily. So, I turned to my very caring wife to do the deed while I turned to look away in disdain. She mercifully agreed to give it a try. Well, that worked about once. I jumped like a skittish six-year-old; she handed the needle to me and never looked back. While I'm not too fond of the shots, I and my tender belly became somewhat callous to the daily routine

Chapter 13
Trials & Tribulations

*A cancer is not simply a lung cancer.
It doesn't simply have a certain kind of appearance
under the microscope or a certain behavior, but it also has
a set of changes in the genes or in the molecules that
modify gene behavior that allows us to categorize cancers
in ways that is very useful in thinking about new ways to
control cancer by prevention and treatment.*
—Harold E Varmus

* * * * * * * *

It was a cold, blustery January morning as we packed up our car with an overnight bag and numerous oxygen bottles stuck in every nook and cranny we could find. Extremely weak and light-headed, I was really struggling in the harsh cold weather. It was imperative that we not miss the appointment in Columbus and risk not getting into the Alectinib Clinical Trial.

Columbus, Ohio, approximately one hundred miles east, was usually a leisurely drive through the countryside, but the ensuing snowstorm changed everything. I had a 9 a.m. Monday morning appointment, so with the blowing snow and twenty-degree temperature, we decided it prudent that we leave a day early and find a hotel near the hospital.

The following morning, we were thrilled to be in Columbus as we looked out at the snow-covered surroundings and a car encased in ice. I awoke extremely weak, particularly in the legs. My only memory of last night was blacking out and collapsing against the wall. The previous day of travel had been particularly arduous. The snow and ice-covered roads made for treacherous driving and frayed nerves.

My anxiety level was quite high as Connie dropped me off at the front door of the James Cancer Center, where I wrestled with the oxygen bottle on my way to the registration desk. The need for oxygen was a new experience for me and one I in no way relished. A bit embarrassed and feeling like a feeble old man, the tubes and canisters were a real pain in the derriere.

As we made our way to the floor and exam room where the study team for Alectinib was located, I was relieved to know they had oxygen connections, thus eliminating the need for any canisters. A nurse from the study team welcomed us and, after a brief chat, began the entry process of the weigh-in, blood pressure, pulse, etc. During the weigh-in, I wondered aloud if being on oxygen would prevent me from getting into the study and was relieved when she assured me it would not be a factor.

Next, the study coordinator came in, sat with us, and shared the essentials, or as often said in the Midwest, "nuts and bolts" of the clinical trial. She explained that I would need a baseline MRI and CT, a washout period from Crizotinib of one week. Visits would be weekly during the first cycle and then evolve into every three weeks, all very similar to my previous Crizotinib trial. The coordinator then gave me registration forms to complete and sign as she left the room to begin scheduling my scans for the study.

The doctor entered next, carrying all the paperwork we had sent in advance, indicating all was in order as he welcomed us to the James Cancer Center. While extremely friendly, I was a little taken aback by learning he was a neophyte to the clinical trial. Throughout our conversation, he seemed to be asking more questions than I and it certainly surprised me when he said they currently did not have anyone enrolled in the study. All of this did not come to me as a total surprise, for I had been one of Dr. Shaw's first patients in the Crizotinib study and realized targeted drugs were definitely on the cutting edge. Hence the small numbers could be understandable. Nevertheless, the young doctor was enthusiastic. I would give him that, and I was equally excited about moving on to the next best second-generation ALK drug.

The doctor exited his chair, shook my hand and welcomed me into the Alectinib clinical trial. On leaving, he indicated the study coordinator would be back in a few minutes with a complete schedule of scans and appointments. I sat back with the first relaxed smile I had for a while, relaxed with the thought I was about to begin a new journey on a new targeted drug. It was renewed hope that I would be getting a second-generation targeted drug that showed promise for the same quality of life I had enjoyed over the past four-plus years on Crizotinib.

* * * * *

After waiting for at least thirty minutes in the exam room, sitting on a very uncomfortable straight metal chair, I might add. My patience was getting the best of me. I was tired, sore, and irritated with the long, unexplained wait. Finally, the study coordinator returned, "Uh, I think we have a problem." I looked up, stunned; I couldn't imagine what she was about to say. Apparently, she and the doctor took a closer look at the medical files I had submitted weeks earlier upon their request and just noticed that I had a previous cancer. The coordinator squirmed a bit as she fumbled with words and ever so slowly mumbled, almost imperceptibly, "That disqualifies you from the study." I almost lost it. Remaining as calm as possible, my first question was straightforward, "What are you talking about?" I could not believe what I was hearing. I had just driven one hundred miles through a snowstorm the previous night and spent over four hours in their facility in preparation for the study, and now they tell me I didn't qualify. She had no answers; they obviously had not done their homework. I asked to see the doctor, who then returned to the room very humbled and apologetic but without any recourse. When I pushed the issue, he agreed to take my situation to the drug company's review board and said he would get back to me in a couple of days. That sounded much like the "don't call me, I'll call you" scenario, but I realized my options were limited by that time.

Needless to say, we left the James Cancer Center with a nasty taste in our mouths. With the snow howling and me exhausted and unable to do anything but sleep, my wife had the unenviable task of getting us home. Yet get us home she did, one hundred miles through a driving snowstorm, navigating in and around snow drifts, and finally clearing the final hurdle of our snowbound farm lane. I was never so happy to arrive home. We both struggled through the biting cold air to get me and my oxygen bottles into the house, where I again collapsed on the sofa in total exhaustion. I never knew how debilitating the need for oxygen could be. I had never been so weak and exhausted as I was at that time in my life.

The following day came with a call from the doctor at the James Cancer Center to let me know what I had already assumed he would say; the drug company was unwilling to make an exception. Having been around clinical trials for a while, I had heard others talk of an alternative possibility called "compassionate care," a treatment option where a patient would be accepted into a clinical trial on a case-by-case basis upon the request and direction of a clinical trial physician. When asked about the compassionate care option, my question was met with hesitation, then deafening silence on the doctor's end of the phone, and I knew our conversation was about to end.

Being a novice in the cancer community at the time, I accepted his lack of concern and turned to my "rock" of support, Dr. Shaw. Knowing what I know now, the doctor's refusal at the James would have been challenged, as I would have pursued access to the trial much more aggressively. Now with my longevity/experience in and around the cancer community, I have found a vast array of sources to assist. One example, Pfizer has put together a very beneficial link entitled "Compassionate Use and Expanded Access."

If, by chance, the reader detected a bit of frustration in my experience at the James Cancer Center, please note that in no way am I being critical of the James as a cancer center. Rather, I have read and heard by word of mouth many very positive experiences. I simply did not have a favorable experience with a specific clinical trial staff.

Lastly, be aggressive and don't take no for an answer when looking into access to a clinical trial. I learned about compassionate access from an individual who worked in clinical trials with a thoracic oncologist: if you are deemed not eligible to enroll in a particular trial, push the principal investigator and the research coordinator to contact the sponsor to make an exception. Even if the doctor/coordinator says the sponsor doesn't make exceptions, push them to ask the sponsor for a waiver. It requires more work on their part, but if they draft the request properly, it may open the door to a drug that isn't otherwise available.

*****

Not a broken man with what I had just been dealt, but I must admit I was very disappointed and disheartened. Yet this setback was wholly different from previous times when dealing with a severe cancer setback. Previously, I did not know where to turn or to whom. This time I knew exactly what to do, for I had one ace up my sleeve, and that was Dr. Alice Shaw.

A call that same day to Dr. Shaw brought a prompt return call, and we immediately began to explore the second-generation targeted drugs that would be best for me. Two particular drugs seemed to be a possibility for me: LDK, soon to be on the market, and Ariad 26113 (Brigatinib), currently in a clinical trial in Boston under Dr. Shaw's supervision. Both required a washout period and most importantly, I needed to be off of oxygen. Therefore Dr. Shaw stated my immediate task was to improve my health and get off the oxygen. Reminding me that I was just days past a very severe blood clot, still had some fluids in my lungs, and was recovering from a severe bout with pneumonia.

My desire to get off oxygen was monumental; I made getting rid of the oxygen tubes and bottles priority number one. In the meantime, numerous doctor appointments kept me busy, with my local doctor ordering an X-ray to check the dissolving of blood clots and fluid in my lungs. Also ordered was an ultrasound of my legs to ensure there were no other blood clots. At the same time, 93% was the magical number to get me off oxygen.

*****

January 14th was the "get out of jail free" date as I rid myself of those nasty oxygen tubes and bottles and gained a new respect for those poor souls forever tied to that unrelenting burden.

The same day, having received my new freedom "from the bottles," I received a call from Dr. Shaw concerning my enrollment in a new clinical trial. Of the two options, I had chosen Ariad 26113, feeling it best fit my immediate need, whereas LDK was awaiting FDA approval and not immediately available. I was not interested in an extended time without an ALK second-generation drug. Dr. Shaw had received all copies of my doctor reports updating her on my condition and had made the preliminary arrangements needed for me to enroll in the Ariad study.

Three days after agreeing with Dr. Shaw that Ariad 26113 (Brigatinib) was the preferred second-generation drug best suited for me, she had me preliminarily enrolled, and a timeline was being developed. Penny, the scheduler, would call me about my first appointments in Boston at the end of January. My wife was now hustling to find rooms at Beacon Hill for the days scheduled in Boston for tests and evaluations.

It was quick; I appreciated the promptness with which Dr. Shaw got me into the study. Ask any person living with cancer what one of the most challenging aspects of dealing with their cancer is, and I'll bet "waiting" would be at the top of the list. Nothing, I mean nothing, can be as excruciating as waiting for a CT/ MRI scan or the nerve-racking wait for results. Called "scanxiety" in the cancer community, it is a feeling of total helplessness and dread beginning days before the scan, if not weeks, and not ending until you receive the report interpreted by your trusted physician. If you have ever been in that situation as a patient, I'm sure you would be nodding your head in agreement.

Back in Boston, just a month after the radiation of my brain following surgery, I was excited to be enrolling in the second-generation Ariad 26113 clinical trial. I hoped this clinical trial would prevent any future brain Mets and lead to a good long run with an excellent quality of life.

I was feeling a bit like the old pro returning to the locker room for another season. I strolled into MGH on that January 27th morning in 2014, confident but with some trepidation about what the future held for me. I was met with a bit of a surprise early on as I checked in at the desk with David, the friendly receptionist. He informed me that Dr. Shaw was out of town and I would be seeing another doctor. It was always a little disappointing when I didn't get to see Dr. Shaw, yet I had come to learn and accept that you have to share when you have the best doctor in the country.

*****

David and I go back to my first introduction to the daunting world of targeted drugs and clinical trials. With his incredible photographic memory, David greets every patient who walks through the door just as he greeted me with a big "Hello, Bill," followed by a gigantic Kenyan smile. I would guess I have walked through those doors at least fifty times in the past six years, and never once did he forget my name or that smile! It's seemingly impossible to explain the feeling you have as an individual living with cancer to walk through a door with the fears and anxieties of the world of cancer and be greeted like that. A dollar amount cannot be placed on that wonderful greeting and smile.

* * * * *

I understood that a meeting with the doctor and a quick physical, followed by meeting the various team members, was the standard mode of operation when beginning a clinical trial. After blood work, we were taken to the exam room to meet the doctor and the rest of the team. As we sat in the exam room waiting for the doctor, Connie gave me a puzzled look and whispered that the doctor's name looked familiar. I shrugged my shoulders in a so-what manner; we had seen various doctors at MGH over our four-plus years. No, this was different; this doctor goes way back. Connie believed this was the doctor I went to see for my second opinion in NYC. No way! I thought as I shook my head, but she was pretty sure, and Connie had a really good memory for detail. She found his name in our address book, and it wasn't but a minute before he came waltzing into the exam room. Getting up out of my chair, I put out my hand and said, "Hello, Chris, how are you; do you remember me?" His smiling face turned to a questioning one as he shook my hand, and I could tell he had no idea who I was and certainly no reason to remember me. I smiled, told him my name, and teasingly finished, "You told me I would be dead in two years; that was almost six years ago." My wife gave me a kick, and I quickly let him know that I in no way held any animosity towards him, that actually, I had at the time appreciated his candor back in 2007. As we began the physical for the clinical trial, he went on to share how he got to MGH, saying, "This is the place to be for lung cancer research." I certainly could attest to that. We finished our surprise reunion by signing the consent forms to start the clinical trial.

I went on to meet the rest of the team as each individual shared how they would be working with me: Penny, EKG and scheduling my scans/appointments; Lisa, research nurse, dispensing the drug (28 days = one cycle); Jen, nurse practitioner, who explained that Ariad 26113 consisted of three 30 milligram tablets once a day (this dose would double after the first week), no food two hours prior or after. Our questions were answered, physical passed, papers signed, and the date set for me to start cycle 1. Fortunately, they were able to use my recent scans as a baseline. I had said goodbye to Xalkori the night before. The "washout period" (time between drugs) would only be three days. There had been a great deal of talk in the "targeted drug" community concerning the length of the washout period. I was happy with the brief washout timeline and was ready and anxious to begin.

Finished for the day, I was ready for some fresh air, so we decided to walk back to the Beacon House, stopping off at the Hill Tavern, our favorite place in Boston, for clam chowder. The Beacon House, our lodging for the next four weeks, was an ideal location while involved in a clinical trial due to its relatively close proximity. Five or six blocks from MGH makes for a reasonably easy trip between the two locations. The only hidden challenge (and I would not call it hidden) is the unforgiving Beacon Hill itself. My overall weak condition would undoubtedly be challenged over the next few weeks by the infamous Beacon Hill.

*****

Day 1 Ariad 26113. The first day of a clinical trial is always a big day, and mine was that and more, as I was told to plan on a full eight-hour day. Beginning with 8:30 a.m. blood work, my first day was packed full as I talked with Dr. Shaw and the entire study team, along with regular blood work and EKGs. The second day became a little less hectic but still very structured, with a great deal of monitoring. Dosing of my Ariad 26113 drug in the form of three pills taken once a day was the central theme and would become the center of my universe for hopefully a good long run. There was concern early on in the study about the dosage amount. Dr. Shaw was concerned enough that she started me off at half dose and was particularly watchful of me, to the point she even called me at my lodging the first evening. (A side note: the concern about AP 26113 wasn't so much the dosage amount but the risk of early and severe respiratory symptoms. A very unusual toxicity unique to AP 26113, but which can be mitigated by taking a lower dose, which is what I was started on.)

After the first two days of extremely close monitoring, I was given a little more freedom as the team handed me a week's supply of the study drug and said, "Enjoy, but stay in touch." The CTs taken by the study team showed a slow but constant reduction of my blood clot, and I could concur because of my gradual increase in strength and stamina. Connie and I decided to take advantage of "free" time and began to explore a cold January Boston that we found to be quite charming. Walks on the Boston Commons and a rather embarrassing failed attempt at ice skating on the Frog Pond were memorable. To my total surprise and disgust, my ankles were like fish as they flopped around like a pair of guppies struggling in a muddy country pond.

The subsequent weekly visits were uneventful, and I was getting stronger by the day. While they had doubled my dose, the Ariad drug continued to be very tolerable, giving us the greatest of freedom to do some real exploring. The well marked Freedom Trail led us off our beloved Boston Commons to some great historical landmarks throughout the city, followed by a much-anticipated Boston Celtics game. Next was a long-awaited road trip to Lake Placid, NY, and a breathtaking bobsled ride down one of their famed 1980 Winter Olympic sled runs filled our days. A stopover in Brattleboro, VT, to visit special friends we had met at the Hope Lodge finished a road trip to remember. By the end of February, we were into Cycle 2, and I was doing well enough that the study team dispensed a month's supply of the Ariad study drug and pointed me west towards the Buckeye State; we were more than ready to spend some time at home with family and friends.

My run on the Ariad study began well in Boston and continued smoothly with monthly visits that included blood work, doctor visits, EKGs, and dispensing of the Ariad drug. Bimonthly visits were similar with the addition of CT and MRI scans. The scans always brought with them a certain level of anxiety, and while I learned to deal with the stress, it never went away. I alleviated a large amount of the stress over time by persuading "the powers that be" early on to eliminate the putrid contrast before my CT. After a severe reaction that literally had me quivering uncontrollably on the scan table, they also did away with my CT intravenous contrast.

Chapter 14
Scanxiety & Travel

"Doctor, did the MRI reveal anything?"
"Yes, you're claustrophobic!"
—Author Unknown

* * * * * * * *

I would like to share this lighthearted poem by Sam McBride, a fellow ALK patient.

"I am going for my scans this morning and I thought I would write a little jingle to cheer you and myself up on this last day of the week. Sung to the tune of School Days, for all of those old enough to remember that tune:

I call it "Scan Days": Scan Days, Scan days, dear old lovely scan days, they poke you and prod you and fill you with dye, they put you in a room so cold you will cry.

You are run through a tube that is not very wide, in a gown so flimsy it barely covers your pride, The tube clangs and it whizzes and takes pictures, inside.

Finally, the whizzing and the clanging ends and you think to yourself Hallelujah, at last, I am done. Then you hear the nurse say: see you back in three months hon! Scan days, scan days dear old lovely scan days!"
–Sam McBride

While I never believed there was anything in my makeup or up-bringing that resembled adversity to machines. That all changed with my diagnosis of cancer. Looking back, I had no recollection of that fear manifesting itself. There was a time in my youth that put me on a machine: a tractor, truck, automobile, etc., and I was one happy young man. Time spent crawling under, over, or even in my old '56 Chevy were some of the best times of my life. In later years, it was purchasing an old '77 Argosy Airstream, restoring it to its glory, and traveling the Alcan Highway and the back roads of America.

Now things had changed. Cancer had crept into my life, bring-ing along such baggage as chemo that evolved into X-rays and an assortment of more powerful scanning machines. My aversion to these scanning machines began from a simple dislike, an inconvenience if you will, to evolve into an absolute hatred of those monstrosities of the medical world.

Following are reflections of my feelings and observations of my interaction with the many, many encounters I have had with the scanning machines and the people who operate them.

Not knowing exactly when my aversion to scans started, I speculate that it may have begun to raise its ugly head with Pet/CT scans at the Indianapolis hospital. For some unknown reason, the Indianapolis hospital called their scans Pet/ CT scans.

While generally, I have been reasonably aware of what was being done to my body, a person living with cancer is much more at the mercy of the doctor and surrounding medical staff than they would care to be. My first inkling that all was not well came during what I thought would be a routine scan when my left arm, receiving the infusion (dye), began to enlarge at the location where the needle entered my arm. At first, just a small discomfort with a slight rise in the skin rapidly evolved into an enormous grapefruit-like lump with a great deal more pain.

A quick shout-out to the young tech brought him scurrying in, and with a concerned look on his surprised face, he quickly removed the needle. A bit embarrassed, he meekly mumbled something to the effect that the needle was not in properly, which was obvious. I shared my agreement and displeasure with him simultaneously with a raised eyebrow frown.

With the above incident ingrained in my mind and the terrible experience I had incurred while struggling with the dangerous, potent drug OxyContin and its negative effect on my ability to endure confining spaces, it was obvious that scans and I were never to be friends again.

Although I joked about my aversion to scans, my years of involvement with clinical trials had caused me to accept the inevitable and deal with the regular scanning regimen. Overcoming the need for OxyContin and a medicine (Lorazepam) taken a short time before, the scanning process became the norm.

*****

I came across this wonderful explanation of "Scan Anxiety" described by a fellow ALK patient on the ALK-positive website by Jeffery Sturm. Jeff is an exceptional writer with a gift for putting words in a very colorful way that expresses what many individuals living with cancer see and feel.

Carcinoma Commentaries

3/14/2021

The Fear

Cancer, the big C. Perhaps the most fear-inducing of all words, particularly when it occurs with your name attached to it. The cold shocking terror of that first diagnosis never seems to go away, but lurks there in the shadows during the waiting times in-between. Sometimes the fear sleeps, and relative normalcy allows for brighter days amid surges of appreciation, love, and gratitude. But then it's time for blood tests, scans, and waiting for results. Scanxiety, operating along a spectrum of angst ranging from unmitigated four-in-the-morning cold-sweating dread, to at best, a dry-mouthed twisting of the innards amidst mumbled imprecations to please let it be ok this time. The worst fear, of the fear itself, springs up out of nowhere, has nowhere to go, and leaves no place to hide. There are many ways to stuff it down, push it out, cover it up, busy-body it away, rationalize, anesthetize, project, and deflect it. Anything to temper the feral sense that mortality itself is threatened, that the invader within carries the possibility of doom, and that there is no escape. Fear is the worst part of the cancer odyssey, and nobody talks about it. We hold it in a quiet place and soldier on, bravely battle, courageously fight. For the most part it's ours alone. Doctors don't address it. Family needs us to be strong. Friends can only hear so much.

But we are not alone. We have this place to share our fears with others who really get it. Maybe that will help a little. Maybe a lot. How do we deal with the burden of fear and make this journey a little easier? Can we start a conversation about this please?

My concern over the high number of CT scans has never diminished. Equally, I am not alone in my concern over receiving large amounts of radiation from scans. A large number of individuals in the cancer community have expressed this concern on many platforms. With the concern over scan radiation, there is, it seems, an obvious "elephant in the room," presenting an extremely difficult question that patients of clinical trials must weigh as they battle their particular cancer. The question, simply put, is the clinical trial drug worth the risk of radiation?

Historically, most individuals diagnosed with stage IV lung cancer were called "terminal." Therefore, the accepted belief was why not choose scan radiation since the terminal patient will likely die long before the radiation can cause damage. But now there is a "new sheriff" in town; that sheriff is called Targeted Drugs, and some now refer to stage IV cancer as a "chronic disease" rather than terminal due to the extended time targeted drugs have added to a person's life while living with cancer. As highlighted in my book, I can attest to the success of the new "sheriff" and speak firsthand; I am currently on my second Targeted Drug, approaching my eighth anniversary since being diagnosed with stage IV lung cancer.

* * * * *

The real challenge came for me with the Magnetic Resonance Imaging (MRI) machine, known by many patients as simply the "tube." To me, there was a much darker side to the MRI, for I found it similar to a claustrophobic coffin. Earlier in my book, I discussed the challenges with the pain medication OxyContin. It had escalated my fear of confined places, and while on OxyContin, any confining space was "no-go" territory. Knowing I had been off the painkiller for six years, I assumed that time of my life was gone; I was wrong. Thankfully, with the help of a little pill called Lorazepam, a great deal of "willpower," and, believe this or not, a mirror, I managed to survive the forty-five minutes of stressful confinement.

Happily, some kind and ingenious individual had devised a "why didn't I think of that idea" that made my life in the MRI machine at least manageable. A mirror, yes, a mirror! I could not believe it until I actually used one, but the simple act of putting a mirror on the headpiece used by the patient made all the difference in the world. Please don't ask me to explain it, but it worked for many other patients with claustrophobic issues and me. Lying in that tube, when I opened my eyes and looked in the mirror, I could see outside, not the confinement within the tube. I know it sounds crazy, but it worked for me.

The mirror, not a standard component of most MRI scanning machines, was, when used, attached to the patient's headgear. As mentioned, I had a high degree of anxiety when placed headfirst into the narrow, enclosed cave-like tube, to the point of having to take medication to calm me for the forced imprisonment. As an aside, on my most recent journey into the tube, the tech casually shared in passing something to the effect she was not sure where she had placed the mirror and asked nonchalantly if that would be a problem. Just wanting to get the ordeal over and assuming with the large number of MRIs I had previously experienced, I quickly said, "Yes, just get this over." With that said, the technician walked out and began my head-first immersion into the tube. As my nose passed within one-quarter of an inch of the inner wall, my claustrophobia was rekindled, triggering my hand on the panic button and a vocal "whoa." This sent the tech scrambling into the next room, where she quickly found the mirror and my tranquility restored.

My experience when walking into an MRI room had a terrible dead sound, the sound of walking into a tomb. I once shared this observation with a female patient, and I got a "Shut up, you're scaring me to death." Obviously, I would not say that anymore because the last thing I wanted to do was have some friends, or anyone, walking into an image room thinking a morbid thought.

I had been thinking about my scans on the drive to Boston and woke up the following morning with scans on my mind. The thought of scan results is always somewhere lingering in the spaces of the mind and comes to the forefront as "scanxiety." Over the past years, I had become somewhat accustomed to the anxiety but never completely immune. I found myself picking up on the smallest physical ailments and suspecting something was amiss.

Now I don't know what has come over me and why I don't have the scan anxiety I once had. Honestly, I would not swear to anyone the next time I go into an MRI machine that I may not scream like a newborn baby, but as I sat in my easy chair typing this chapter, I had no anxiety about the MRI scans. Let me assure you; I would still ask for a "wide body" machine whenever possible!

*****

During this period of what I called "healthy bliss," the Ariad clinical trial drug was very "body-friendly," with minor diarrhea being the only side effect of any consequence. The bouts of diarrhea could usually be controlled with diet and the little blue Imodium tablets. Dare I say without being too graphic? There was the occasional frantic search and sprint to the nearest facility that made my life just that much more interesting.

Traveling fever kicked into high gear with the easiness of the clinical trial drug Ariad. In talking with Dr. Shaw, there were no significant restrictions, including travel overseas. Though I can't speak for others living with cancer, I'm relatively confident many of us are plagued with the places-not-visited syndrome, often referred to by the aged travelers as a "bucket list." I may be one of the worst at lamenting not getting to the many places I had always dreamed of, and let me assure you, that list is endless.

In the four previous years, Xalkori had brought me back to the edge of normalcy and enabled us to do some traveling. Now with Ariad, I found a targeted drug that would allow Connie and me to continue to not only hit the open road but also hit the open sky.

With the proverbial "sky's the limit" attitude, I now had the enthusiasm of a modern-day Marco Polo. We scanned the world map for overseas destinations I had dreamed of, but with my cancer diagnosis, I assumed it would never happen. I was ecstatic: places like The Great Wall of China, Machu Picchu, and the Seine River to the Beaches of Normandy. All felt the bottom of our loafers as we wandered the ancient lands of the Far East to the sands of Normandy.

EXPLORING THE RUINS OF MACHU PICCHU, PERU

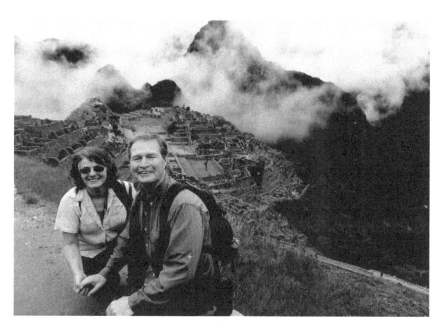

* * * * *

Travel Tips

I had been asked on numerous occasions if it was difficult to travel as a person living with cancer. My answer is not as difficult as one might think and definitely not so challenging as to keep a person living with cancer at home. I would suggest some considerations for anyone traveling with targeted drugs. Be sure your medication is clearly marked and separate in your carry-on, allowing easy access for customs. We have traveled to five continents and have never had the first problem with customs if drugs are visible and easy to access. Also, be cognizant of having and maintaining a proper temperature/environment for your drugs; a small cooler worked well for us. One big concern we had not given much thought to was the medication schedule and the various time zones we would be traveling through, making sure to continue taking the drugs at the proper intervals. My wife was my timekeeper (a watch with multiple alarms was very handy), and I know she and I were challenged as we tried to look at time zones, maintaining the critical time gap between each dose. We also found packing a bag of appropriate snacks beneficial as a supplement used with medications on long excursions.

Wherever we traveled, good drinking water was a constant concern for all travelers, and of course, hydration is particularly critical for an individual living with cancer. We found tour companies were typically very diligent about supplying the water or making sure it was available to purchase. We also stayed away from any water poured into a cup (including ice), and that included water for brushing our teeth. Here are a few more tips to be equally important for travel in general and those living with cancer. We were warned against eating raw vegetables or from salad bars and consuming raw and uncooked foods. We have always carried individual packets of hand wipes for an assortment of sanitary needs, such as airplane trays, hotel room tables, restrooms, etc.

Those who have traveled overseas, particularly in any third-world country, know well that sanitation can be a genuine concern, especially if one's immune system is compromised, as it is for anyone living with cancer. If a third-world country is on your itinerary, I highly recommend checking with your local doctor or hospital about going to a travel clinic. That was recommended for our trip to East Africa for our planned safari. It was highly beneficial. The doctor was very knowledgeable about Africa, and we went away with all the shots and paperwork needed. Finally, when traveling, there are many challenges compounded with age and all that comes with the need to have a port-a-potty at your beck and call.

Chapter 15
Progression? Stable? Responsive?

The devil whispered in my ear.
"You're not strong enough to withstand the storm."
Today I whispered in the devil's ear "I am the storm."
—Posted anonymously

* * * * * * * *

Two years into my very amicable time on the Ariad 26113 (Brigatinib) study drug, the powers that be thought it was time for a name, thus deciding on Brigatinib. The clinical trial drug that had allowed me the freedom to hike, bike, and basically gallivant like a kid around the world was growing up and now had a name of its own. What may surprise some, the naming of the second-generation drug was quite a noteworthy event for the ALK community. Yes, only in the world of cancer could the naming of a cancer drug be considered an event. But an event it was, for those in the know are very cognizant of the fact that the naming of a clinical trial drug is one more very critical step to FDA approval.

Routine became the norm in our travel to Boston and MGH as the months rolled by in a somewhat monotonous manner. Typically looked upon by many individuals in a negative light, the word "routine" in the cancer world certainly finds a place of acceptance. A routine schedule is often seen as a positive for those living with cancer as they march through the vast array of mind-numbing procedures. Dauntlessly accepting the countless pokes and pricks with little more than a wince, holding nothing but the assurance of their attending physician that there would be the proverbial "light at the end of the tunnel."

Routine even seeped into the very depths of our clinical trial team. My wife and I were saddened to see the personnel changes in the Brigatinib study team as members filtered off to other avenues on their varied career paths. But others replaced them and were just as talented and friendly, ready to provide the needed comfort, knowledge, and support.

With my months of bliss represented in the many stable CT and MRI scans, my wife and I monitored the scan reports. We carefully reviewed them before filing the reports away, a valued tip from a friend, who good-naturedly referred to himself as a "well-worn" person living with cancer. We quickly discovered a language/terminology existed within those lead-plated rooms the technicians labored in that needed to be deciphered before getting anything useful from a radiology report. With time, a person living with cancer typically learns three basic words to identify their cancer status within the reports: progression, stable, or responsive. One can go as deeply into learning the ins and outs of a radiology report as one would like, but without the assistance of a qualified physician at your side, it would be a daunting, if not impossible, task. On a somewhat humorous note, I had on occasion overheard discussions in the various waiting rooms between individuals expounding on the various terms of a radiology report; all I can say relating to that is, patient, beware of the waiting room radiologist!

Even while I enjoyed the first two years on Brigatinib and the outstandingly stable bi-monthly CT and MRI reports, the inevitable would have to raise its ugly head. And even with all my talk and outward show of confidence, one lingering thought was always in the back of my mind when I walked into that cold, sterile image room. "Is this the day my cancer comes back?" As mentioned early on, there was even a period in which the scans were so clear of any signs of recurrence that my plea for extended time between scans was surprisingly accommodated, with an increase to four-month intervals. We were now making the sojourn to Boston on a schedule allowing my blood work to be completed at my local health care center in my hometown of Versailles, Ohio. What a difference. Now instead of a 1,700-mile round trip to Boston, it was a half-mile drive, or often if the weather allowed, a 20-minute walk or quick five-minute bike ride to the health center.

As we entered the third year of my uneventful run on Brigatinib, there began to be the ever-increasing signs in my perfect world of routine and stable scans that something may be amiss. Seeds of questions were beginning to take root and while not totally justified, they annoyingly lingered.

More of the same, as my subsequent two scans covering four months indicated that it looked like the possibility of growth, but no conclusive evidence would call for immediate action. Meeting and talking with Dr. Shaw and Dr. Shih after each MRI scan seemed to be the same conversation; if there was progression in the brain, it was minimal and very slow. I certainly appreciated being involved in "what comes next" conversations with the doctors, secure in the knowledge these two bright ladies were always one step ahead of the game and would have the answers when need-ed. Our conversations about ALK inhibitors became more realistic and definitive as it appeared the possibility of some changes was coming, albeit slowly.

*****

My suspicion of something amiss became more than a gut feeling as Dr. Shaw and my radiation oncologist Dr. Shih believed there could be some change when looking closely at my May 2016 report. Two of the best doctors I know agreed about seeing some type of change on my MRI but could not and would not stipulate precisely what it was. They talked of possibilities besides cancer, including different MRI machines, radiologist opinions, residual brain radiation side effects, radiologist technique, an anomaly, etc. They agreed that a wait-and-see approach would be our "modus operandi" until the following scan. I certainly understood some of the hesitation and confusion as the doctors described what they saw on the scans as inconclusive. Also in the mix was the very de-tailed but difficult-to-understand radiology report that was shared with us by the doctors. As stated previously, radiology reports are often difficult to read and sometimes very noncommittal, as with the May report.

On each visit to MGH for scans, there would be a scheduled doctor's visit coinciding with my clinical trial and the dispensing of medication, EKG, and other study protocol requirements. On those scheduled visits with both doctors, we discussed what they saw on the scans and the radiology report. Also included in the visit would be a cognitive memory test, balance test, facial expression test, and other methods used by the two doctors to evaluate my phys-ical and mental capabilities. There appeared to be no mental or physical health concern on my part that would give cause for the doctors to look beyond the scans for any abnormality. Of course, there would be those in my world of friends who know me very well and would happily expound on my abnormalities for as long as one would be willing to listen.

Always a positive throughout the years of scans, and I do mean years over nine at this point, has been that my lung cancer appears to be very slow growing. That has always been my one "lifeline" from the very, very beginning. During the darkest times when the terrible chemos ravaged my body, I harkened back to the secure thought of the time-wasting "sluggishness" of my cancer.

*****

Big change on floor 7, the MGH thoracic cancer center. David was gone, the ever-so-friendly receptionist at the desk who always remembered everyone's name with the greatest Kenyan smile this side of the Atlantic. He had been promoted to a higher position on the ninth floor (no pun intended). Tears were flowing in the phlebotomy lab when I asked if they missed him, a rhetorical question to which I knew the answer, but in no way did I expect the drama that accompanied their response. To say they missed David was a gigantic understatement. The absence of David could be seen in the chaos of the waiting room, which, during David's time, was a sea of tranquility.

Our arrival into Bean Town had become so commonplace that we jokingly replied on occasions when asked where we were from, "Boston" was our response with a wink and smile. On the last count, we had made our way to Boston and MGH well over 75 times. Not complaining, for Boston and its people have been good to us. As guests in their city, many individuals had extended gestures of kindness, like the guy in the local tavern who overheard my cancer story and offered me tickets to a Red Sox game. Or a helping hand like the shuttle bus driver "hooking me up" with his buddy when I needed a good spare tire (to replace our 50-mile donut tire) to get home. And we can't forget the jovial MTA conductor helping us buy our first tickets, then handing each of us a Charlie Card for future use. But the Boston winters! Now that's another story.

Snow was nary a concern on our July arrival in Boston for scans and checkup; this trip brought with it a bit of trepidation, as my previous scan showed the slight possibilities of some change. And while it had not kept me up at night (the aforementioned dilemma lingering in the back of my mind), the thought of cancer recurrence had been messing with me.

However, I had found a diversion that definitely was working its magic to allow my mind to think of far more pleasant thoughts. Yes, my health again allowed me the opportunity to travel overseas, as I figured this was the time for that long dreamed of African safari. Hopefully, if the timing/date worked out, we would be in the Maasai Mara National Reserve of Kenya for a glimpse of the Great Migration.

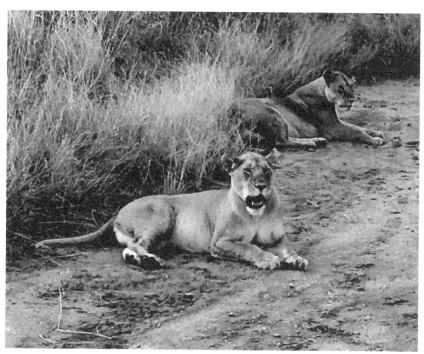

LIONS ON MAASAI MARA KENYA, AFRICA

When traveling overseas during my cancer journey, I always tried to arrange our overseas flight date with a scheduled clinical trial visit—knowing that the trial study visits were regimen protocol and needed to adhere to a very strict timeline. It was simply an attempt on my part to make lemonade out of lemons by combining a somewhat negative experience of a cancer visit with a vacation. I need to add a note of caution here. With my stage IV cancer, we had found it prudent to purchase travel insurance with pre-existing conditions and sometimes included the "cancel for any reason" option for obvious reasons.

*****

The July MRI report continued the discussion about changes. This time both doctors were adding that, if indeed it was cancer, it was too early for any brain radiation treatment. This was followed by a discussion of just how it could be treated. Whole brain radiation was ruled out but considered was Intensity Modulated Radiation Treatment (IMRT) or divided targeted radiation. Brought into the conversation for the first time was a discussion about the options I would have if I had progression in my brain. I would take the following options home to mull over, research, and discuss. The first option to consider would be the other second-generation ALK inhibitors currently on the market, Alectinib and Ceritinib. A check with insurance coverage was suggested. An increase in dosage of my current drug, second-generation Brigatinib, could be considered, as well as the third-generation ALK inhibitor Lorlatinib, currently on a clinical trial. Finally, to be considered was Radiation versus Drugs.

It was pretty obvious when reading over my radiology report that the reason for the possible changes in my treatment plan being discussed had been stimulated by my MRI radiology report:

"Minimal enlargement of three small enhancing foci... favoring treatment effect, through slowly progressing metastases are not entirely excluded."

While my last two MRIs had not been the sterile clean reports I would have liked, as a so-called "battle-scarred soldier" of the cancer battles, I realized there were more battles to be fought, and in no way was I looking to send up the white flag.

I also knew from experience that it was not wise to rush into battle but rather allow my fellow soldiers and their commanders (Dr. Shaw and Dr. Shih) time to prepare a battle plan before the all-out assault on my cancer. This was in reference to my early years of cancer and my rushing into various ineffective chemotherapies. In reality, I had to admit that the chemotherapies may have caused more harm than benefit.

So, following a reassuring meeting with both doctors that my cancer was stable throughout my body (except for my brain, where there was just too much inconsistency to be conclusive). We would again reevaluate in two months. I had a lot to think about, particularly with the possible changes in the future and the options I had. Thankful for the options, for I remembered vividly the time early on in my cancer journey when there were none. We left Boston and headed to Long Island for a visit with our grandkids in preparation for our vacation flight out of JFK. I was secure in the feeling that, while I had hurdles to face in my future, I was in the best hands. With the blessings of the doctors and entire clinical trial team, who I might add were "over the top" jealous, Connie and I laced up our boots, put on our safari hats, and headed out the door to the dark continent, Africa.

"Out of Africa" is the movie that motivated and inspired our dream of visiting the "Dark Continent." Now let me ask the reader, how could anyone not go to Africa after viewing Robert Redford and Meryl Streep soaring through the beautiful crystal blue skies of the Maasai Mara plains in their 1937 open-air cockpit Biplane? The amazing aerial cinematography of the movie was all the impetus we needed to research, plan, and carry out such a trip. Please don't ask my wife about all the shots required to visit Africa! It would not surprise anyone that our first stop after landing in Nairobi, Kenya, was a stopover at the home of Karen Blixen, author of "Out of Africa," published in 1937, a true story that the movie portrayed. Walking around and through the original home (now a museum) was a walk through a place frozen in time. One only needed to close their eyes to hear and feel the presence of Karen Blixen, Kamante, her house boy, multiple guests, and of course, Denis Finch-Hatton. This home/museum visit was just an interlude to our safari across the Maasai Mara with close-up views of the "Big 9," namely, Lion, Elephant, Rhino, Leopard, Buffalo, Cheetah, Hippo, Giraffe, Zebra. It was topped off with a balloon ride, giving the traveler a unique view of the boundless African plains at sunrise.

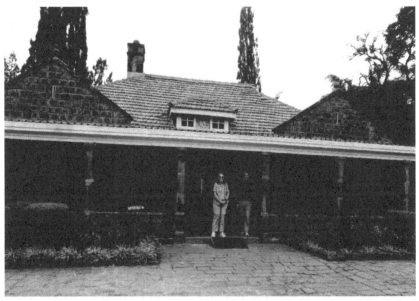

HOME OF KAREN BLIXEN, AUTHOR OF *OUT OF AFRICA*, NAIROBI, KENYA

*****

Returning home, I had seriously considered Alectinib for the simple reason that it had been approved and was on the market. It also had an early reputation as a very viable second-generation drug. Word in the cancer community was that it was working exceptionally well, particularly in crossing the blood-brain barrier in an attempt to eradicate brain Mets. As was commonly accepted in the targeted drug community, the two drugs, Alectinib and Ceritinib, had been considered the standard second line of attack in the progression of fighting lung cancer. Both were on the market at the time and after checking with my insurance plan, both would be available as specialty medications. This meant authorization would be required along with ordering the medication monthly from a specialty pharmacy at a tier-three cost.

After a conversation with Dr. Shaw, she strongly believed that Lorlatinib would be my best choice. She felt that staying with a second-generation drug would be a lateral move. Remember, I had been on the second-generation Brigatinib and had an excellent two-and-a-half-year run. All reports about Lorlatinib had been good, so with Dr. Shaw's recommendation; I was leaning heavily towards starting a new clinical trial with the third-generation drug, Lorlatinib.

At my November study trial visit, I was a little disappointed that Dr. Shaw was out of town. I guess it was just a comfort thing, for I had made up my mind, with just a few items to be clarified. To be honest, there was no reason for any disappointment. Our questions were answered satisfactorily by the attending doctor, who had the consent form to be used by enrollees in the new Phase II Lorlatinib Clinical Trial. The doctor explained he was not looking for us to commit at that moment, and actually, they were not quite ready to begin enrolling patients. We could take the consent form home to review closely and call Dr. Shaw with our decision.

We thanked him for his information and shared that we would be out of town for a week or so, actually out of the country. I asked if that would be a problem. He assured us there was no big rush; they were not enrolling patients at the moment. He told us to enjoy our trip to Iceland and contact Dr. Shaw on our return.

We continued to make lemonade out of lemons. The quick five-day trip from JFK to Iceland that we had scheduled to coincide with the November trial visit was enjoyable. The small island was a delight. And although, after our three-hour wait in a cold sub-zero temperature, the Northern Lights show was not the spectacular display we had hoped to see. We were entertained by a "junior" display of the northern sky on our bus ride back to the city. As we enjoyed the rugged beauty of the "Land of Fire and Ice" and its wonderfully friendly people, my mind was not far from home and the Lorlatinib study trial.

As I contemplated my third targeted ALK inhibitor and the 10th anniversary of my cancer diagnosis, this would be an appropriate time to address the notion of being "cancer-free." Oh, how I would hope that to be true, but for anyone who knows much about lung cancer, the one universal fact is that at this time, lung cancer is a terminal disease. I am amazed at the number of people whom I meet, friends and acquaintances, that have the misunderstanding of my cancer being cured. They see me on the street, and often, if it has been a long time, like a year or more, I'll get that "second take," usually followed by a hesitant, "Well, you look good; how you doing?" Then, depending on how close a friendship we had previously, the personal questions would come.

Many, if not most, of my friends knew I had been diagnosed with stage IV lung cancer. I did not hide it; they read it in the newspapers, saw it on local news, and actually on the national news as I shared it with the world. So understandably, when they see me around ten years later, and I'm still walking above ground, they automatically believe that I had been cured. All I could say to them without entering the realm of spirituality would be I was blessed, and I mean blessed. Then, depending on their level of interest and sincerity, I share my success with the various targeted drugs and ALK inhibitors that have been introduced into the world of cancer. With the new ALK inhibitors, the incredibly debilitating harshness of side effects usually associated with cancer treatments has been greatly reduced, thus allowing the individual living with cancer the ability to carry on an active lifestyle, along with looking and feeling good. Hence the bewildered looks and scratched heads were understandable.

We decided on the new study trial and put a call into MGH. Numerous challenges delayed our contacting Dr. Shaw to discuss specifics. Of particular importance were study trial dates.

Chapter 16
Lorlatinib
A New Dog to the Fight

*"Cancer can take away all of my physical abilities.
It cannot touch my mind, it cannot touch my heart,
and it cannot touch my soul."*
—Jim Valvano

* * * * * * * *

D r. Shaw had brought another "new dog to the fight" at our early November 2016 checkup, with the news she would be sponsoring a new Phase II study for the targeted drug Lorlatinib.

Music to my ears, for this, was a third-generation drug on a promising clinical trial that had closed at the end of August. Fortunately for me, Dr. Shaw was starting a new study, as shared:

(Research consent form,2016) Protocol Title: A Phase II study of Lorlatinib (pf 06463922 in advance ALK and ROS1 rearranged NSCLC with CNS metastasis in the absence of measurable extracranial lesions.

It's expected that about 30 people will take part in this research study.

All participants will receive Lorlatinib. Lorlatinib is made by the Pharmaceutical Company Pfizer. Lorlatinib targets the abnormal ALK or ROS1 proteins in your cancer cells. Lorlatinib has been tested in other research studies and results show that the medicine may help to control the growth of your cancer even after it has spread to the central nervous system (CNS). The CNS is a term used to refer to the brain and spinal cord, including the lining of the brain and spinal cord which is called the meninges. When cancer has spread to the CNS, it is called CNS metastasis.

In this study, Pfizer is trying to determine whether Lorlatinib is effective in controlling the growth of cancer cells after they have spread to the CNS. Another purpose of this study is to determine why the cancer cells that have spread to your CNS have continued to grow despite treatment with other drugs. For this reason, blood samples will be collected as part of this study to assess the DNA released by your cancer cells into your blood when the cells travel to other sites in your body.

Screening: After signing the consent form, the screening will include: medical history, physical exam, performance status, tumor assessment, blood samples, urine sample, EKG, ALK, or ROS1 confirmation.

Following the successful screening and a seven-day washout period, I would receive the study drug: 4 tablets (25 mg each) taken once a day and a monthly drug diary (to be completed daily). Each treatment cycle would last 21 days. During each cycle, I would be taking the study drug Lorlatinib once per day.

Risks or discomforts of the research study? One risk was that the drug would not help treat the disease. Common side effects: increase in cholesterol; damage to nerves in hands, arms, feet, or legs; causing tingling or numbness; mood changes, including irritability; slowing of speech; fatigue; nausea; and abnormal liver function; constipation and weight gain. Also possible: high blood sugar, decrease in red blood cell count, changes in blood pressure, changes in kidney function, pancreatitis, and rash.

The Lorlatinib Phase II clinical trial seemed to be a perfect fit for me, as one of the main focuses of the trial involved previous ALK patients whose cancer had metastasized to the brain. There were also complications, as in any clinical trial; this one would deal with the protocol required of a doctor and trial team visit every three weeks. In addition, we would be required to spend the first two weeks in Boston at the start of the trial for an array of activities, including meeting with the trial team for dosing, EKG and blood work, etc., as stated above. Also mentioned was the exposure to scans. While a challenge, Connie and I had become accustomed to extended stays in Boston.

* * * * *

Oh, what a difference two weeks could make. I was now on I-80 driving painfully east to Boston, a miserable man. My face was ablaze; I looked like I had just walked out of a bar-room fight and had gotten the worst of it. Actually, one would guess that I had not gotten a punch in! And it was not just the look in the mirror that brought pain to my body; the red blotches on my skin had me itching and scratching like a dog with fleas.

I had no clue where this rash came from, but why now, just as we were headed east to Boston, I did not know. My mind raced, thinking back over the last few days of the specific things I had done that may have caused this unknown rash to break out, not only on my face and head but also on my hands and arms.

Could my local YMCA pool water possibly be the culprit? Was it something I ate or where I had been that would have caused me such an aggressive rash? Nothing came to mind, nothing except that I had a few days earlier quit taking my study drug Brigatinib. Although a coincidence, I didn't think that the mere stopping of the drug would cause such a rash. Well, if there were a bright spot in this entire dilemma, it would be that I was headed in the right direction and the best place to be with a health issue, MGH!

My arrival in Boston was the scratchiest drive I have had in the past eight years. We would be staying north of the city on this trip. The Beacon House, with its excellent proximity to MGH, was unavailable. With the extremely high cost of lodging in the vicinity, we found something much more affordable in the town of Woburn. Only ten miles north, someone like myself from a small village typically would think nothing of it; but country boy beware, there was something in Boston they called city traffic. Need I say more? Yet, we had stayed in this northern lodging numerous times and learned to get up early to beat the traffic if there was such a thing as beating Boston traffic.

My screening day for the Lorlatinib clinical trial was the following day, and I cannot express the urgency I felt. My rash had gotten much worse over the last couple of days of driving, and I could not wait to get to MGH for some possible relief.

An "Oh my," with a hand over their mouth and a ghost-like look was the typical reaction as I circulated through the various hallways and waiting rooms. I finally landed at my destination point for the screening. Jen, the nurse practitioner, was the first on the team to meet me. Of course, being the health professional she was, her reaction to my red-ravaged face was controlled except for the grit of her teeth as she took a close look. "What's this all about?" was basically what I expected to hear, and my response was a very defeated, "I don't have a clue."

The long-awaited suggestions soon began: lotions of all sorts, coconut oil? But sadly, she too was stumped as to the cause. Hence a specific recommendation did not follow. Possible causes, such as sun poisoning, which I knew was painful and certainly irritated the rash, didn't seem that likely, for I had not been in the sun for any extended time. I wondered out loud if the drug I had just stopped, "cold turkey," a few days before could have anything to do with the rash; it was such a coincidence for this rash to occur so close to my quitting the drug. Jen didn't think so and concluded by saying she would talk with Dr. Shaw and thought the use of a hydrocortisone cream might be helpful but cautioned me to use it sparingly.

On the positive side, having a rash would not deter my entrance into the clinical trial. Thus, Jen started with a detailed outline of what would be involved. Having experienced two previous clinical trials, we were pretty knowledgeable, so it was just a matter of filling us in on the specifics of the Lorlatinib study. I would need to be off my previous drug, Brigatinib, for seven days, called a washout period, basically for clinical trial purposes to ensure the last drug is out of the system. Knowing this in advance, I had stopped the drug three days before I left home so we could start the new ALK drug immediately at the end of the seven days.

Another specific issue of the study was the typical rise in cholesterol levels that tended to follow when taking Lorlatinib, so I would be given a statin to help lower my cholesterol as a preventative. Weight gain was another issue identified to be watched, as several trial patients had experienced weight gains of up to twenty pounds. Now that was one big drawback. Weight had not been a concern of mine, but it should have been particularly during my forties, the "middle years," so now I tended to watch my diet more carefully.

Finally, there seemed to be genuine concern over emotional temperament with this study drug. So, the team directed attention to Connie and me about monitoring irritability. I certainly detected a wily smirk on Connie's face as she would be involved in monitoring my temperament. I wondered to myself how in the world I was possibly going to be able to drive down the highway anywhere in the United States and not be involved in some level of "increased temperament!"

With a signed consent form in hand, making me the second enrollee, Jen excused herself, sharing that she would be talking with Dr. Shaw about the mysterious rash. Next in the room was the study team, the same study team I had with Brigatinib, so the transition from my previous study drug to my new study drug, Lorlatinib, would be with the same individuals, which certainly made for an easy transition. Blood work was completed earlier, along with a satisfactory EKG. I was free to go for the weekend, returning on Monday to begin the study with the first dose of Lorlatinib. Our first task after leaving the hospital was a drive to a pharmacy to hopefully relieve my rash, which seemed to worsen by the hour.

* * * * *

Monday, Nov. 21, 2016, was yet another milestone in my cancer journey, for I was about to begin my third ALK inhibitor drug, Lorlatinib, in a phase II clinical trial. It had been quite a trip to this point. Right at ten years since my lung cancer diagnosis and a little over eight years of being on the life-saving ALK Targeted drugs. It had been quite a ride with staggering emergency room visits, brain surgery, radiation, the many pricks of the needles, and the countless anxiety-filled hours in the MRI machine affectionately known by yours truly as "the tube."

The dose of four pills was without fanfare, as I recalled the dosing at my first clinical trial with the targeted drug Crizotinib some eight years earlier and thought how far we had come. My anxiety level at that time was off the chart; I was dying. Yes, that sounds dramatic, but I "WAS" dying. Every doctor I had seen for the first two and a half years had pumped their poison into me and then sent me on my way home to die, along with a somewhat somber message of, "You had best make plans."

Different was my third clinical trial. Oh, the anxiety was still present. For now, the cancer was in my brain and possibly growing again; and if not Lorlatinib, what? A caveat of a sort was the timeline for eating, including food restrictions. Basically, there were none. For the past three years, I was, or should I say, my wife was making sure that I did not ingest any food two hours before nor two hours after taking my study drug pills. While I improved with time, I often forgot the time intervals; therefore, staying on a regimented schedule was preferred. It would not have happened without my wife and her trusty alarm-ringing watch.

On Monday's arrival, Jen shared she had talked with Dr. Shaw extensively about my rash, and she believed stopping my previous study drug was directly connected. She further suggested I get a hydrocortisone cream immediately and use it sparingly on my face. Jen also asked permission to take pictures of my hideous face, which I reluctantly agreed to, as she intended to share them with Dr. Shaw.

Required by the study protocol to return in a week, we decided to forgo a two-day drive home to turn around in two days and drive back to Boston. So, the rest of the week was spent hanging around Boston pool halls and assorted backroom bars… just kidding. The rest of the week was pretty dull, to be honest. I was miserable, so to push my rash dilemma out of my mind, we ventured into Boston daily for various activities, including catching the matinee movie "Hacksaw Ridge." We also visited the Boston Commons, where they were trucking in their famous Christmas tree fresh from Nova Scotia. The tree had quite a unique history. A local proudly shared how since 1971, the tree had been a gift to the people of Boston from the people of Nova Scotia in thanks for their assistance after the 1917 Halifax explosion. Having an entire week and feeling lousy, I thought taking another bus tour of the city would be relaxing and comfortable. It was meant to be somewhat of a time killer, but it turned out to be very enjoyable even though we had taken a similar tour years earlier. It is interesting how much the tours differ with the various guides.

My meeting with Dr. Shaw came one week after my initial dose, and she seemed pleased with everything. Regarding the rash, it appeared to be turning the corner, but I was to keep using the hydrocortisone cream. We were headed home with a quick return in just two short weeks for the start of cycle 2. That return trip was pretty much routine; again, the checkup was with Jen. We were all happy my rash was vastly improved, and my blood work results were good. There seemed to be some swelling in both my ankles, not severe, but something to keep an eye on. One thought was the possible long automobile rides to Boston. The one noticeable, out of an otherwise routine checkup, was a weight gain of twelve pounds. "AAUGH!" as Charlie Brown would say. It was then a quick goodbye and back to Ohio, anticipating my first scans thirty-eight days since switching to the new study drug Lorlatinib.

* * * * *

Following a weekend visit with family, a relatively short drive from Long Island to Boston got us in the night before my scans. It would be both a long day and an early one, with a 7:15 a.m. report to Yawkey 6. It was good to be in the night before. I liked to be well rested, for the fasting blood work, CT, and MRI could be somewhat exhausting. This would be the first CT and MRI five-plus weeks after enrolling in the Lorlatinib clinical trial, so there was a bit more anxiety than I had experienced for a while.

The following day we met with Dr. Shaw to review the scan results and, if need be, make adjustments to the treatment plan. My blood work looked good. Next came the CT scan results, which were stable and had been for a very long time, years in fact. Scans are typically taken of my chest and abdomen, which includes the lung where we assume my cancer originated. So, we were very relieved that the cancer in my chest remained stable and monitored the surrounding area as a precaution.

To my dismay, a few years back, lung cancer had metastasized to my brain, hence the surgery followed by radiation. Now the third-generation ALK Inhibitor Lorlatinib will hopefully penetrate the brain-blood barrier, eradicating any cancer that may be present. Dr. Shaw shared that the MRI brain scan showed the cancer to be stable. A little disappointed, I had hoped it would have, in layman's terms, "knocked it back" a little. I tried to read a bit of optimism or pessimism in Dr. Shaw's voice, but even though I had been a patient of hers for eight years, she was too much of a professional to let a thought she did not want to disclose slip out.

The word "enhancement" was used in the radiology report, a vague term: an enhancement could be anything, a shadow from the machine to actual cancer, so definitely not anything on which to make a decision. There was little to no change with what we saw on the MRI scan. Dr. Shaw wanted to get the advice of her cohort Dr. Shih, the radiation oncologist, who was better trained in reading a radiology scan but happened to be out of town. Her advice was to continue on the same drug and dosage and see what the next set of scans looked like in six weeks, and she would call after talking to Dr. Shih. True to her word, Dr. Shaw was on the phone with me at home, sharing that Dr. Shih concurred that there appeared to be a possible change. They both agreed that we wait for the next scan results and hopefully would have a significant enough change to decide on treatment.

Visits to Boston for the Lorlatinib clinical trial were pretty much run-of-the-mill. Until my clinical trial nurse practitioner casually asked how things were going, I responded somewhat animatedly, "My hair, I'm losing my hair," as I ran my hands through my ever-increasingly thin hair. I then shared how my home shower floor looked like sheep shearing time on an Australian Outback ranch. The nurse was seemingly unfazed by my animated tirade as I continued my mournful dialogue of how I watched large quantities of my thinning locks circle the shower floor on the way to the drain. She just smiled, giving me no indication that this was a possible side effect and perhaps would moderate in time. Rather, with a sly smile, my friendly practitioner said softly, "Bill, you know that older men tend to lose their hair with years." We all had a good laugh; sadly, I dare say, at my expense. In all seriousness, there is something quite traumatizing about one losing their hair. To an individual living with cancer, it is like cancer has taken my energy, strength, and appetite; does it also have to take my pride? Enough already!

*****

While driving to Boston had been a challenge over the years, the real highlight was the opportunity to visit with my daughter and her family living on Long Island, NY. Often as possible, we combined a trip to Boston with a stopover on Long Island for a visit with my daughter, her husband, and, of course, our three wonderful grandchildren. A chance to see the prettiest little dancer in New York and the best two young hockey players skate their hearts out was the best medicine a person living with stage IV lung cancer could have. Therefore, we always made a concerted effort to correlate the dates of my trial checkups/scans with activities within my daughter's household and the upcoming Thanksgiving and Christmas holidays.

Fortunately, I had a doctor who was very aware of the importance of family and especially mindful of doing everything in her power to help schedule the quagmire of doctor and family visits. That said, when we finally connected and confirmed our commitment to the new clinical trial, Dr. Shaw was more than obliging in comparing schedules and calendars. That ensured I could be in Boston for scans and office visits, allowing for a holiday trip to Long Island. This was an extra step, maybe not taken by all doctors, but one I hope to be true of most.

So, our next trip back to Boston for the Lorlatinib trial would be by way of Long Island, NY. We had arranged my doctor's visit and scans in conjunction with a trip to NY for the holidays. We arrived at my daughter's home on Christmas morning in 2016 to a house that, regardless of how much picking up took place, still had that wonderful look and remnants of Santa making his arrival on Christmas Eve. Of course, Grandpa and Grandma could not be outdone by Jolly Ol' St. Nick, so we stumbled in lugging our gifts of plenty. Nothing like a houseful of loved ones and wide-eyed kids rocking and rolling throughout to keep a grandpa's mind off scans and tests in the next few days.

Of course, a trip to New York would not be complete without a trip to the city and a tour of the 9/11 Memorial and the Freedom

Tower. I had shared with my daughter my wish to visit the Memorial and the tower, and she was making it happen. The following day we packed up the crew, drove to the train station, boarded the Long Island Railroad to Grand Central; we hopped the subway to the towers. Oh, if only it could be that easy. Grandpa had forgotten about his crew having one 8-year-old, a 6-year-old, and a very energetic 4-year-old.

On top of that, as we prepared to leave, the 8yr old "NYC tycoon" came walking downstairs dressed for the part in his First Communion suit, complete with tie. Somewhat stunned, his mother questioned the suit and immediately got a very reasonable answer. Since the grandkids had been promised a visit to their parent's workplace, both attorneys in the city, he certainly needed to dress the part. A hesitant smile from his mom brought a "What the heck, let the kid do it" from his grandpa as we proceeded out the door and on to what I was sure to be a great adventure.

An adventure it was and memories by the dozens as we watched the grandkids follow the path of their parents to work, to experience the trains, subways, and yes, the chance to sit at their mom and dad's desks. I was profoundly moved; no, not by the office desks, but rather by the fabulous work completed by the designers and builders of the 9/11 Memorial. Equally impressive, if not more so, was the massive interior of the building. The displays were breathtaking and heartbreaking, a "don't miss" stop on any visit to the "Big Apple."

* * * * *

A hard-blowing February nor'easter was somewhat of a surprise as Connie, and I plowed through the Pocono Mountains of eastern Pennsylvania into New York on our next monthly trip to Boston. We typically checked the weather forecast before our travels, and my wife, in particular, was usually very attuned to the weather; somehow, we missed this one. The mixture of ice and blowing snow made for one of the more "white-knuckled" drives I had experienced in the past eight years of driving to Boston. As our front-wheel drive SUV's tires spun and struggled to keep us heading in a northeastern direction on I-84, my mind kept returning to the four-wheel drive F-150 I regrettably left parked at home in the garage. The pickup truck had been discussed briefly; the forecast we had seen called for the storm to go further north, making the need for a four-wheel drive unnecessary, or so we thought. Three to four hours behind schedule, we literally "slid" into Boston, weary and exhausted yet extremely happy to have arrived safely without any dings, dents, or wrecker calls.

If there was a positive to the lengthy and challenging drive, it would be that it took my mind off the following day's CT and MRI scans scheduled, along with the foreseeable hassle involved in getting to the off-campus facility at the Chelsea location. I had previously expressed my dislike of the MRI, so when told by my scheduler that all machines at MGH were booked and I would now need to go to the Chelsea location, a challenging drive across town, my disdain escalated another notch. But, to the credit of my scheduler, she had arranged transportation from MGH, significantly relieving my stress of negotiating the back streets of Boston.

Moving my scans to Chelsea rekindled previous questions regarding radiation levels in the different CT and MRI machines at the various MGH locations. While very friendly, typically, when talking with the individual technicians at the two separate locations and asking about radiation levels, I never seemed to get direct answers. When asking about a specific CT machine and the amount of radiation or comparisons, I usually received a rather vague reply. My last discussion with a tech at Chelsea was quite different; rather than getting the typical vague answer, he provided me with a definite "I don't know!" I actually appreciated his honesty when asked why my MRI time was 15 minutes less than an MRI at MGH. I shared that my time in the MRI had always been the same length at MGH and now was 15 minutes shorter at Chelsea. His "I don't know" came with a questionable clarification that all the computers use the same program. Thus, time in the MRI should be the same regardless of building. Ah, the unknowns of science?

While the drive over was somewhat of a hassle, I appreciated the friendliness of the staff at Chelsea. I got a particularly deep chuckle from the Jamaican technician whose first words to me after a name and number identification were, "How's your vein?" Taken aback, for I had never been asked that question in my ten-plus years of getting an IV, I fired back with a smile, "How's your ability to find one?" This resulted in a returned smile, an excellent needle stick, and blood draw.

The following day when stepping onto the scale in the doc's office, to my chagrin, the new drug Lorlatinib was packing pounds on me. Early on, Dr. Shaw had shared I would probably have some water retention, hopefully leveling off around twenty pounds. Oh, man, that's like telling those on board the Titanic to throw the musicians overboard, and it should level off. I finished by warning Dr. Shaw not to think about leaving a granola bar near me, or my ravenous appetite would devour it before she saw her next patient.

*****

A little disappointed with the absence of Dr. Shaw at my clinical trial checkup; another stable scan report had me feeling comfortable. Coupled with the "calm" demeanor of Jen, the nurse practitioner, who shared that they again believed a wait-and-see was best for me at the time. I had become somewhat immune to the fact that cancer could be growing in my brain. This knowledge that it was slow growing and the uncertainty of progression by the doctors seemed to ease the stress somewhat.

Radiology report: *Impression: Stable examination. No evidence of progressive metastatic disease. Stable foci of nodular enhancement within the left inferior cerebellar hemisphere, just lateral to a previously radiated left celebellar metastasis, not significantly changed since 10/31/2016. Stable post-operative and post-treatment findings related to prior resection of left occipital lobe metastasis and radiation to a right occipital lobe metastasis. No findings to suggest local tumor recurrence.*

Another bright note that truly came out of the blue from the clinical trial team was the decision I would no longer need to visit every month but would change to every other month. Wow! Talk about a surprise! I had just talked with Jen about reducing the number of visits, and she had not given me much hope for a change anytime soon. While the change from one month to two months may not sound like much of a difference, as I have stated previously, while looking at the big picture, that meant half the number of trips to Boston, which was huge.

Chapter 17
Life on Lorlatinib

"I don't have a choice as to my "new" normal, so I do what I can do to continue to find enjoyment and fulfillment in life."
—Ed Steger

* * * * * * * *

I trust my readers have gotten a sense of my sometimes over-the-top obsession with the effort of incorporating "fun" travel experiences to and from cancer treatments. Most family and friends already knew that I loved to travel. It can be said that I have a passion for travel. My wife would state it quite differently, simply, "Bill is a travel 'nut'!" This is true, and as I have often shared, my infatuation with travel is the responsibility of my introduction to the National Geographic magazine by my memorable fifth-grade classroom teacher, Mr. George.

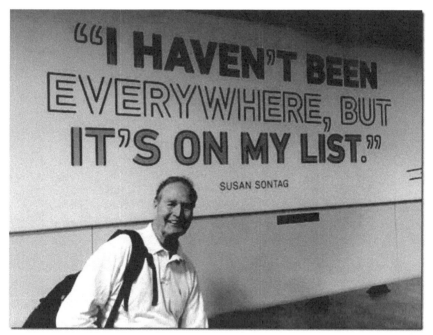

BILL AT JFK INTERNATIONAL AIRPORT, DREAMING OF FUTURE TRAVELS

So it is not surprising that I am constantly scrutinizing the latest travel brochures and websites for the best travel deals of the week. I always considered how it would best fit into a trip to Boston for checkups and then a drive to Long Island with often a flight out of JFK for worlds unknown.

On the other end of the spectrum was my friendly neighbor's quizzing comment, "How the hell do you do it?" when inquiring about how I handled all the driving back and forth to Boston for the various clinical trials (three clinical trials and counting). I returned with, "Do you know what you just asked?" I looked at him for quite a while to let it sink in. I followed his puzzled look with, "You just asked me why I fight so hard to stay alive." He replied, "Really, you're still getting treated for that? I thought you were cured." He and his wife seemed unaware they were talking and standing next to an individual living with stage IV terminal lung cancer.

I was certainly relieved to put all thoughts of lung cancer to the back of my mind and focus on our upcoming trip to the Middle East country of Egypt, another one of those trips I had dreamed of since my boyhood days of seeing the world through the pages of the National Geographic magazine. This trip would be the first time I had traveled out of the country while taking the newly prescribed drug Lorlatinib and a test of my ability to travel on a flight that required sitting for long periods of time.

Before flying to Cairo, the flight to Egypt was a challenging eleven hours, with a four-hour layover in Jeddah, Saudi Arabia. The obvious challenge would be the initial eleven-hour flight; although I had purchased my ticket well in advance for an aisle seat when I arrived at my seat upon boarding, it was a window seat, to my dismay. The smiling but not so accommodating Saudi stewardess was less than understanding when I shared that I had some serious issues with blood clots and needed the ability to get up and walk on occasion. She casually mentioned that six aisle seats were available and would check into them when possible. My eyes brightened as I thanked her. As the other passengers climbed aboard, I watched closely to see if the stewardess had been successful in acquiring me an aisle seat. Sadly, it appeared she was making little or no effort. When I finally got her attention, the boarding process had been completed, and no aisle seats were available.

Upon our arrival in Egypt, my ankles and legs were noticeably swollen. The inability to get up and walk during the eleven-hour flight had been my downfall. You can bet on our return trip; I used the compression socks and swore to myself that not having an aisle seat to allow me access to frequent walks would not happen again. I had dealt with swollen ankles and legs with my first ALK inhibitor, Crizotinib, but seemingly to a lesser degree. Time would tell, but it looked as though I would have to be much more proactive regarding long-distance travel.

Aside from the challenges of long flights and swollen legs, travel with the Lorlatinib drug had been hassle-free. Our most significant health scare of the trip came from an unlikely source. The night before our scheduled flight out of JFK, our daughter's son was vomiting profusely throughout the night with a nasty stomach virus. As one can imagine, Connie and I quietly slunk out of the house the following morning to the awaiting car service for our ride to JFK, praying we had not picked up the virus.

Our worries over a stomach virus had been unwarranted. As we arrived in the land of "sand, sultans, and camels," we were both healthy, though a bit tired, stiff-legged, and, of course, my swollen ankles. I was hopeful that the answer would be raised legs and many sightseeing walks.

*****

The following day we awoke in the shadow of the pyramids, where we rode the camels before embarking on a four-day Nile River cruise through the Valley of the Kings. Elevation of my legs at night and daily sightseeing tours in the Valley of the Kings had brought relief and near normalcy to my once swollen legs. Once again, putting an exclamation point on the fact that there is life with stage IV cancer! ALK-IES (an acronym for anaplastic lymphoma kinase patients), in particular, have been given a second lease on life and a firm belief of mine that it not be squandered.

I would be remiss if I left our trip to Egypt without sharing a humorous, albeit scary, camel adventure. To set the stage, as we ventured toward the Pyramids on our tour bus, my excitement was running at a fever pitch. The long-awaited adventure of seeing the Pyramids up close, a lifelong dream, was about to happen. Our Egyptian guide laid out our schedule and activities as the bus scurried through the dirty, dusty city of Cairo toward the Pyramids on the outskirts of the capital. She was emphatic that we follow her instructions regarding the many vendors surrounding the Pyramids and to be particularly wary of the notorious camel ride vendors.

Like many heavily visited tourist attractions, the Pyramids had the unscrupulous pickpocket and other scam artists. But what set the Pyramids apart from all of the other tourist destinations had to be what some would call "camel jockeys," a derogatory term. I came to fondly call them "camel dudes." Now to say these individuals were persistent is like saying the desert has sand. They just never give up on trying to get you on top of their long-legged creatures.

Along with the firm and clear warning about the aggressive "camel dudes," our guide shared that the company had arranged a camel ride for us, which was included in our tour package. She continued that it would be in a much better location, including the Pyramids in the background, and we would have photo opportunities galore. Delaying the camel ride was an obvious no-brainer, and I wondered to myself why she felt the need to repeat the point numerous times as though we were grade school children, a thought that would come back to haunt me, as the reader will soon learn.

My excitement escalated with the occasional glimpse of the Pyramids as we ventured toward them. But it was not until we stepped off the bus and the reality hit me did I realize the unforgettable enormity of those three colossal structures. The Pyramids were everything I thought they would be and so much more. We were able to touch the perfectly carved enormous boulders that are still to this day a mystery as to exactly how they were constructed.

After talking my wife into a long walk around the largest of the Pyramids built for King Khufu and wearing out my Kodak, it was nearing time to return to the bus. A simple task, one would assume, but sadly things began to go amiss. Instead of returning to the bus with my wife, the spirit of Indiana Jones grabbed hold of me with the thought of a few more minutes of exploration. Perhaps even finding that million-dollar photo, aka the holy grail of pictures.

As I strolled towards the bus, passing one of those smiling, innocent looking "camel dudes," I happened to look back casually. I couldn't believe my eyes. That million-dollar picture, the holy grail! There stood the smiling "camel dude" holding the reins to his magnificent camel with the Pyramids in the background and the perfect sunset falling behind the three-thousand-year-old vestige of the Egyptian empire. I spun around with the speed of a cobra and "click," the picture I was sure would be on the front cover of every National Geographic and every coffee table worldwide!

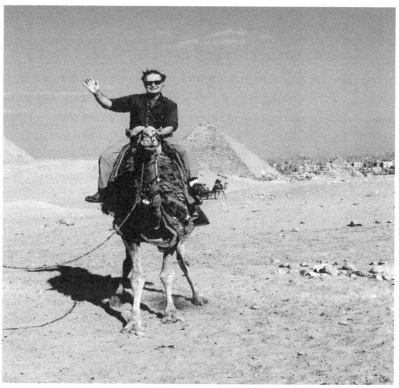

WILD CAMEL RIDE, PYRAMIDS, CAIRO, EGYPT

Oh, it gets better. Ecstatic over my Rembrandt-like creation safely stored in my Kodak, aka smartphone. Yet feeling a bit guilty that the friendly smiling owner of the camel was not reaping any reward, I thought it a kind gesture if I gave the old fellow an innocent tip. How could that be anything but a positive act, right? Well, the old smiling fellow graciously accepted my dollar and, in what I thought to be gratitude, directed me to stand in front of the camel that, in all appearances, seemed to be peacefully resting in the sand. He would then take my picture with the camel and Pyramids in the background.

Can the reader see where this is going? Sadly, my Indiana Jones instinct for treachery was not as acute as it needed to be. When I handed the kind old gentleman my camera phone, he snapped a few pictures and then motioned for me, remember he is talking in Arabic, to sit on the camel lying in the sand for a few pictures. Hesitant, I casually waved him off, indicating there was no need, but he was a persistent "camel dude," I thought, what the heck, just one more picture. What could that hurt? Oh, what a mistake! No sooner did my derriere hit the back of that camel than up he went with the speed of a leopard, but not the gracefulness.

You would understand if you have ever seen a camel get up or perhaps had the unfortunate occasion to be on the back of one as it rose to its feet. The rump rises first causing the person "onboard" to nosedive down at every bit a forty-five-degree angle and, if the occupant aboard is fortunate enough not to be thrown like a missile to the ground, the gangly animal then jumps to his two front feet like the spring of a jack rabbit.

Precisely what happened to me is somewhat of a blur. What I assumed to have happened is that after my posterior hit the camel and the rollercoaster rise of the beast began, all the instincts of survival kicked in as I closed my eyes and hung on for dear life. Seconds later, I could feel the air through my hair as I opened my eyes to the passing of King Khufu's Pyramid.

Now the camel was at a full gallop with me crying out at the top of my lungs "Stop this crazed animal now!"

It all ended abruptly as my still smiling "camel dude" grabbed the reins and brought my Egyptian Steed to a halt. Or so I thought. I was now being approached by a multitude of "camel dudes," all claiming that I owed them for my, get this, "camel ride!" Refusing to pay anyone, anything, for a ride I had not planned to take nor asked to take, I was thankfully rescued from a dozen or more angry "camel dudes" just in the nick of time by a very agitated tour guide. So ended my Indiana Jones escapade at the Pyramids! No million-dollar picture for National Geographic; instead, a heart-pumping camel ride, everlasting memories, and a head-shaking wife as I stepped onto our tour bus. With our Egyptian adventure coming to an end, we bade farewell to the Sphinx; shaking sand from our sandals, we boarded our plane for the long flight home.

*****

If you have been around a patient and caregiver for an extended time, you have undoubtedly noticed the drama that seems to be a constant companion to anyone living with cancer. I am not sure I have all the answers, but I believe it has to do with the weakness of a patient's immune system, identified by the one-step-forward and two-step-backward theme.

This could not be more obvious as I strolled in from our ten-day overseas trip to Egypt, another trip I could only have dreamed of when told ten years earlier I would be dead in two years. I had been diligent with using only bottled water, being watchful of foods, using hand wipes, and avoiding raw vegetables. In other words, I followed the advice of all the experts to stay healthy throughout my travels. Somehow, Connie and I even avoided the very harsh stomach virus that left no one standing in my daughter's family home.

So, one could hope that I would not be penalized too much as we returned home, and I re-entered my normal lifestyle, including the first couple days of yard work and the sorting through ten-plus days of delivered mail. I even felt so good the first couple of days at home that I made the extra effort of going to our local Y, combining a two-mile workout on the elliptical trainer with a half-mile swim in the lap pool.

Then it hit! I awoke with a sinus-plugged head that continued for the next three days, and a tingle in my chest gradually progressed into a deep burning cough that I had not experienced previously. Annoyed more than concerned, I shrugged it off as any thirty-year-old would. The problem was I was not a young thirty-year-old. Rather, I was a sixty-eight-year-old man with stage IV lung cancer who previously had brain surgery leading to a pulmonary aneurysm and should have addressed the issues much sooner. It was painfully evident by the end of the week I needed to get to the doctor. Hastening that decision was a mild rash on my left arm that was quite similar to poison ivy, which after a couple of days of applying Calamine lotion, did not go away. A bright, early Monday morning call got me into the doctor's office. A few thumps on my chest, followed by the stethoscope, necessitated a chest X-ray that indicated a partially deflated lung and a pneumonia diagnosis.

As for the puzzling rash on my arm, that was immediately identified as shingles, which certainly made sense. I remembered how Dr. Shaw had cautioned me about shingles, saying it could be related to stress and how that certainly went hand in hand with cancer. She went so far as to recommend I get a vaccination for it, which I had done. Can I assume it would have been worse if I had not? There was some talk that the vaccination induces the rash; I tend to question that rationale.

On the third day following my doctor's appointment, the nurse called to ask how I was doing. My response was, "Who won the fight?" After an extended amount of silence on the other end of the line, I jokingly continued by sharing that my ribs felt like they had gone fifteen rounds with Sonny Liston. More silence on the other end of the line. She was too young, didn't follow sports, or couldn't have cared less? Which one? Let's pick all three. Not sure what she reported back to the doctor, but I would have loved to have been a mouse in that room.

*****

Back in Boston for my bi-monthly scans, I was happy to have a check on my pneumonia (clearing up nicely) along with my routine checkup. I had the occasion to use the open MRI at MGH on the Chelsea campus for my brain scan. I had been hearing about the new open MRI and was excited about the open concept and anxious to try it. When I first entered the MRI imaging room, there sat a large, beautiful, white gleaming machine with the appearance of being wide open. Like a school kid being told of a snow day, I happily jumped up on the MRI machine, but my joy quickly diminished to a weak smile as my enthusiasm turned to disappointment. While the machine was open on both sides, I was inserted, pizza oven-like, into a very narrow space with my nose again only a micro distance from the inside of the machine. Taking deep, slow breaths, I brought myself down from panic mode to an uneasy/uncomfortable mode. If any consolation, although my head was secured as if in cement, I could see a glimmer of light when I looked with strained eyeballs to my right and left.

A bit disappointed, for I had envisioned an open-space machine very similar to what is used for CT scans. I wondered if the crude mirrors attached to the headpiece used with other MRI machines, which somehow gave me the feeling of openness, was not better.

Interestingly, on our next ride from MGH to Chelsea for my May scans, a doctor, who introduced herself as a radiologist, rode along. She was somewhat chatty for a doctor. At least from my experience, the doctors always seem pretty "close to the vest." In other words, a person usually didn't get much from a doctor other than the facts, no chit-chat. The young female doctor was quite the opposite, asking where we were from and eventually inquiring about my thoughts concerning the new MRI. That certainly got my attention, for I longed to talk with those responsible for decisions concerning the machines. When her questions eventually turned to the MRI machine and what I thought about the new "open" machine, I answered with all the gentleman in me by responding that it was OK, but I had expected it to be much "more open!"

She chuckled and said she had heard that before from patients. Aware of her interest in the MRI machine and particularly a patient's opinion, I shared that what I liked was the mirror attached to the headpiece. To this, she seemed a bit taken aback, which surprised me, for I would have thought many other patients would have agreed and expressed their comfort with the mirror.

Back to Chelsea for more scans, and what do I see? Fish. They now had fish swimming around the MRI imaging room at the Chelsea off-main campus. Now obviously, there were no actual aquatic sea creatures that I have so dramatically alluded to; instead, they had brought in a video.

So, one can imagine my surprise when I climbed up on the MRI machine, lay back, put the earplugs in, and closed my eyes as they clamped the mirrored face mask on. Opening my eyes as they pushed me into the machine was a stingray swimming by; I blinked only to see a hammerhead shark rise out of the sea floor. "A mirror?" I heard the tech mumble as he walked out of the room to start the scan procedure. But what was the mirror showing me? An aquarium, I thought. No, that was not possible. Then I quickly realized they had a TV screen located in line with the mirror on the back wall. Oh, the wonders of science.

Crawling off the table, I took a quick glance at the back of the MRI machine as the tech asked with a smile, "How did you like the view?" I replied with a thumbs-up and a feeble attempt at humor, sharing it could have been better with a little NASCAR on the screen! He got a real chuckle out of that, shaking his head, and I could tell he was searching for a comeback that just wasn't there. Smiling, I let him know I really wasn't a NASCAR fan, but if he could arrange for a Patriots game on the screen this fall, he would have patients fighting for tube time! Another big ear-to-ear grin and a belly-shaking laugh as he escorted me out of the room. I believe I made his day.

* * * * *

On May 20, 2017, back home from my positive checkup and scans in Boston, I was given the green light for our planned Baltic cruise. We were excited to finally get a chance to visit some of the northern nations of this world and a unique opportunity to visit the Evil Empire, Russia!

Flying into Denmark, our visits included the small countries of Finland, Sweden, and Estonia before our much-anticipated stopover in Russia. Connie and I were impressed by Estonia's small country and its people. Immediately departing the ship, we noticed a mom-and-pop bicycle tour company and thought, why not? It was a relatively small country, and we did not have a set itinerary. Best decision we made for the entire cruise, for as we joined the small group of riders, we learned very quickly we had a local guide who possessed a wealth of information. With a big toothy grin, the first words out of his mouth as we began our ride were, "We love President Trump and have paid our NATO dues!" For the next few hours, as we leisurely rode our bikes around their small countryside, he not only pointed out the various sights but told us the inside stories. The guide, a fiftyish native of Estonia, had been required to serve in the Russian army and expounded on his negative time in the military and the Russian occupation. He ended by sharing how happy he and his family were now living in free and independent Estonia.

As an aside, I noticed how fluent the young people were in English and asked a young boy if that was from being taught in school. His response was not what I expected when he shared with a confident smile,

"No, I just watched a lot of American cartoons."

Our quick one-day bus ride into cold and rainy Saint Petersburg, Russia, was very interesting and informative. Sadly highlighted by a stop at the checkpoint as I began the exit process and found the stoic-looking customs officials not very accommodating. To be very blunt, they seemed to be extremely intent on making life very difficult for my return to the ship. To sum up my stressful exit, my thought to my readers would be, "Have you ever seen a Russian smile?"

*****

In October 2017, I celebrated my birthday by, you guessed it, more traveling. This time we were staying within our borders by combining a few National Park trips with a visit to my son and his family in sunny California.

A flight into Seattle found us visiting the Olympic and North Cascades National Parks, followed by a drive south to Redding to visit my son and family. Then it was on to Great Basin, Nevada, for completion of the National Parks in the lower 48.

In November 2017, I celebrated my first year anniversary of the Lorlatinib trial. My check-up could not have been better. The brain MRI had finally shown "Responsive/Stability" after three years of questionable scans.

The holidays would be a celebration.

Chapter 18
Living Life
with Side Effects

"I intend to appreciate, marvel and enjoy
all the time that I have left,
with cancer or without it."
—Saskia Lightstar

* * * * * * * *

As time on my current ALK/TKI, Lorbrena, expanded to over five years, the side effects had some similar aspects as well as some noticeable differences from my previous TKI's, Crizotinib and Brigatinib. Having been one of her first patients on the Lorbrena clinical trial, I asked Dr. Shaw what the side effects would be, and she shared, "It's early in the trial; we're not totally sure."

Following are some of the side effects of Lorbrena that may be expected and have been shared by Dr. Shaw and other Lorbrena patients:

–Fever

–Upper respiratory tract infection --sleep problems

–Cognitive effects (problems with memory or attention)

–Dizziness--muscle, joint, or back pain

–Weight gained

–Diarrhea

–Constipation

–Nausea

–Vomiting

–Tiredness

–Headache

–CNS (Central Nervous System)

CNS symptoms include.

- Impaired concentration, confusion, and abnormal thinking.

- Mood swings, including anxiety, agitation, depression, paranoia (feeling very anxious or nervous), and euphoria (feeling very happy).

- Sleep disturbances, including insomnia, drowsiness, vivid dreaming, and nightmares

- Increase in cholesterol

–Liver and kidney problems

–Hypertension

–Vision changes (such as blurred vision, decreased vision)

–Swelling ankles/feet/hands

–Numbness/tingling of arms/legs

–Speech problems

–Fluid retention (edema)

* * * * *

January 2018. As my Boston check-ups continued on a routine trajectory, "the travel bug" struck again. A brief stay with our Long Island family preceded our next-day flight out of JFK to Australia. A very, very long flight left me sitting on the deck of our cruise ship in Australia, awaiting our next-day departure. I could not help but notice the world-famous Harbor Bridge looming in all its enormity near where we were moored. Said to be the eighth longest spanning-arch bridge in the world and the tallest steel-arch bridge measuring 134m (440 ft) from top to water level, it was indeed an awe-inspiring sight.

I took note of some tiny ant-like creatures moving along the very top of the steel structure and casually asked a passing ship steward what those tiny objects crawling along the top of the bridge were. He gave out a big laugh and said, "Why, Mate, that's some crazy tourist out for a morning stroll!"

Wow, I could not believe it! I had to do that! An hour later, I reluctantly plopped down my two hundred bucks, sat through a safety briefing, and suited up. After some laborious, and need I say unnerving climbing, I found myself waving to Connie on the ship. She could not see "Bill the ant" as he waved. From the top of the Harbor Bridge, I discovered the high-priced ticket and laborious climb well worth the most breathtaking views of Sydney, Australia.

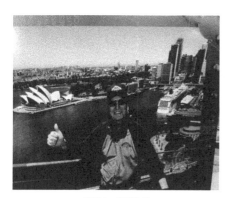

BILL ATOP
HARBOR BRIDGE

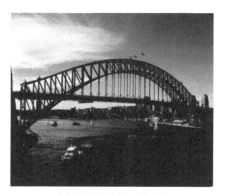

HARBOR BRIDGE
SIDNEY, AUSTRALIA

A travel note: I had arranged our cruise by remembering years back as a bicycle guide; I had asked an older gentleman who had traveled the world what country was his favorite. Without the slightest hesitation, he said, "New Zealand!" Hence, our trip included a cruise to Australia, Tasmania, and, of course, New Zealand.

* * * * *

Back home after a whirlwind cruise of "down under," we were back to reality, attending May birthday parties and graduations. The reality of lung cancer, never far away, raised its ugly head again. I had thought that almost everyone involved with lung cancer was aware of genetic testing. That was until I ran into a friend at a graduation party who told me that the doctors had just diagnosed her husband with lung cancer. Obviously, they were devastated. I then asked if they had discussed testing. She shook her head tentatively, which I took as they had not. The look of bewilderment in her eyes told me she had no idea what to do. I then went into my, "If you don't mind me suggesting mode," to which she replied very emphatically, "Oh, please do!" I advised her to ask the doctor if they had completed a genetic test for mutations; she stated she definitely would.

As the party continued, I happened to observe the couple sitting off to the side of the hall. Their sad eyes told the entire story. They were scared to death. Sitting on a couple of bar stools in the

War Veterans Hall, the couple looked to me as if they were the only color in a room of black and white. A bit later in the evening, I glanced in their direction, and they sadly were still sitting where I had left them. I knew I had to say something, so I walked over to see if I could lift his spirits with some small talk. What I discovered, to my dismay, was he had a small spot on his lung they had been watching for a couple of years and finally did a biopsy, finding it was cancerous. Sadly, they had been "watching" a spot on the lung for two years without doing a biopsy!

* * * * *

July 2018. Boston checkup and review of scans. I had a long talk with Dr. Shaw about the large number of scans and the by-product of so many of them. One concern was about the Gadolinium-Based Contrast Agents (GBCA), which were intravenous drugs used in diagnostic imaging procedures to enhance the quality of magnetic resonance imaging (MRI) or magnetic resonance angiography (MRA). Seeing the enthusiasm and willingness of Dr. Shaw to discuss my feelings and concerns about the MRI process, I thought it would be an opportune time to get some long-inhibited questions answered. A gnawing concern of mine had always been the amount of GBCA I had been accumulating in my body. I had read that the FDA had investigated the use of Gadolinium, and at this time, it showed no specific harm to patients. But there may be long-term effects; hence, they are monitoring patients receiving GBCA for any signs of adverse effects on the body. If there is any relief from anxiety, GBCA is being used in Great Britain with seemingly little concern.

* * * * *

The major difference between Lorlatinib, now known as Lorbrena, and the other ALK Inhibitors I had previously taken has turned out to be very significant, that being the side effect involving the brain.

As I approached my second anniversary on Lorbrena, the one side effect I had not dwelled upon or discussed was the temperament issues associated with Lorbrena. When I first began taking Lorbrena, one of the first questions asked by Dr. Shaw dealt with temperament. Interestingly, she always turned to my wife. It made sense, for she was the person who saw my behavior first-hand.

Not sure if it was a cumulative thing, but I seemed to be having more issues with temperament. It's hard to describe the rationale. What I found to be so aggravating was realizing I was getting angry, which, in turn, made me angrier. Now is that a "mouthful" of nothing, or what? It's as though I'm inside a person that I can't control, really a very unique and sometimes maddening situation.

While I am not an authority on Lorbrena, I do speak as one who has taken the drug going on two years, and it is a drug that penetrates the brain. Hence, it is a potent substance that has effectively prevented a recurrence of my brain Mets. So, continue I will, with continual monitoring of its effects on my mental stability.

Two years into my time on the Lorlatinib Clinical Trial, I lowered my dosage from 100 mg to 75 mg daily, thinking that the decrease might improve my temperament. To be honest, I don't know if it worked. Guess I should be asking Connie. Along with the dosage reduction, I was doing so well we changed visits to every three months, with scans ahead of time at home.

For my fellow Lorlatinib users who may be wondering what Dr. Shaw thought of the reduction, she was all for the reduced dosage! She suggested the possibility when I originally started the trial, believing the dosage was too high.

Oct. 17, 2018, my 70th birthday party, is one way to put cancer on the back burner for a while. Friends all around laughing and smiling; there was nothing better. Extra special was my daughter, who organized the "shindig," flying out from New York with her family. The smiles and giant grins as they were all wearing hats identifying my birthday with "Happy Birthday, Old Man" was priceless.

*****

Increased time between clinical visits from two to three months definitely increased my ability to book overseas travel. Hence, Connie and I booked a trip to the long-desired destination of Israel. What we thought to be just an interesting vacation at booking turned out to be one of our favorite countries visited. Personally, choosing a specific guide when booking a tour was not a practice I had considered, but after our visit and tour to Israel, that all changed; our 10-day tour of "Walking in the Footsteps of Jesus" was an incredible experience. This was all due, in my opinion, to the wonderful guide who showed and shared the story of Jesus as historically factual as possible. Also due, I believe, to the fact our guide was a young man born and raised in Galilee, Israel, and who had an excellent background in archaeology.

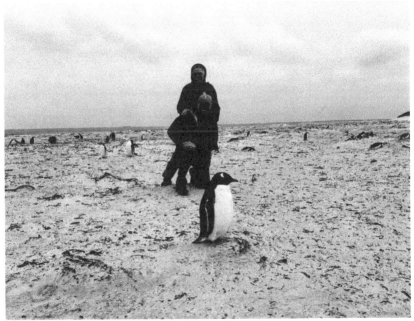

WALKING AMONG THE PENGUINS ON OUR ANTARCTICA CRUISE

February 2019, "Walking with the Penguins, "Yes, you heard me right: an Antarctica cruise, one of those items on the bucket list that I had dreamed of but never really thought was possible. When lung cancer smacked me in the face, the thought of any travel fell to the bottom of the bucket; it was replaced by the very real "battle of my life!" Fortunately, Lorbrena was controlling that battle; hence, the bucket list trip of a lifetime.

Why the Antarctica cruise, you may ask? A dream going back to the first time I picked up the book *"Endurance: Shackleton's Incredible Voyage"*, a riveting story of men getting stranded in the Antarctic and their survival.

*****

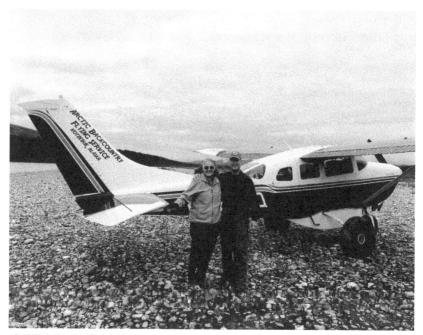

BUSH PLANE RIDE INTO THE GATES OF THE ARCTIC NP, ALASKA

Putting cancer in the proverbial rear-view mirror, my travels continued as I eagerly planned for an Alaskan trip that included bush plane flights into some of Alaska's most remote National Parks. Sadly, as my planning progressed, a very formidable "roadblock" threatened to bring my previously planned flights in

Alaska to a serious and dynamic halt in the form of a major hip replacement. After a year or so of nagging leg pain, a routine visit/checkup to the local doctor discovered that what I thought to be a recurring knee issue turned out to be a serious hip issue. The hip was disintegrating at an alarming rate and had escalated into an urgent need for replacement surgery. The pain was seriously debilitating, enough so that I was ready for immediate surgery. The problem was the doctor's schedule was not ready for me! This dilemma was compounded by the fact that I had already scheduled and paid for a trip that included a flight to Alaska and a couple of bush plane flights into the interior of four different National Parks.

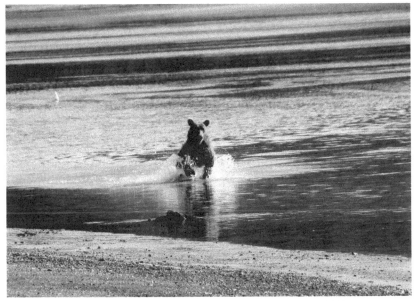

BROWN BEAR FISHING, KATMAI NP, ALASKA

As a side note, hiring a bush plane pilot was not an easy task, particularly if located a couple of thousand miles away in Ohio. Throw in the fact that the bush pilots want their money in advance, and believe me, the Gates of the Arctic, Katmai, Kobuk Valley, and Lake Clark National Parks were not inexpensive flights. For example, my telephone conversation with a bush pilot in Alaska went as follows:

"Hello, my name is Bill Schuette. May I ask the price to have you fly my wife and me into the Gates of the Arctic?" "Sure," the friendly Alaskan bush pilot answered, "Two thousand dollars." Wow! That was not what I was thinking, but before I could think of a response, out of my mouth came, "I don't want to buy the damn plane; I just want to rent it!" A chuckle on the other end of the line rather than a click assured me he had not hung up. With a slightly calmer voice, I asked if he was serious. Needless to say, he was "painfully serious!"

Having made the payments for all four flights in advance, we were north to Alaska with a much lighter wallet regardless of the painful hip I was compelled to drag around for the ten-day trek.

I survived the Alaskan trip, having visited the four National Parks requiring a bush plane and viewing some of the most beautiful scenery Alaska had to offer. But let me tell you, it was at a painful cost as I literally crawled in and out of the planes on numerous occasions. One of my most painful/memorable moments was placing my size-eleven foot "inside" a grizzly bear's footprint as I hobbled out of the plane onto a trail we were to hike. Thinking, what am I to do if we come nose to nose with that bear? My wife didn't seem to have the same concern about the grizzly as I did. She reminded me of the old adage if a grizzly did appear, she need not worry about outrunning the bear; she would only need to outrun me!

*   *   *   *   *

As a person diagnosed with stage IV lung cancer early on, I had the following attitude about many things, "What the hell, this cancer is going to kill me anyway." So, anything involving future decisions was pretty much dismissed, or the term I remember using was "Put on the back burner." That all seemed to change with time as my TKIs (Tyrosine Kinase Inhibitors) seemed to be working better than I had expected, a surprise to me as I believe it was with others throughout the cancer community. As life's longevity seemed a little brighter, I gave pain and long-term suffering a different look. I was now much more proactive at addressing the debilitating issue of pain in my hip.

At my July clinical trial check-up in Boston, while sharing my decision about hip surgery and all that it involved, I questioned whether a surgeon could deny my surgery due to my being diagnosed with stage IV lung cancer. A clinical trial team nurse came out of her seat exclaiming, "No one can stop you from any type of surgery due to your cancer!" That's all the reassurance I needed.

Hip replacement completed; the medical terminology was osteoarthritis with avascular necrosis. The question was, why did I wait so long? After a precautionary one-night stay in the hospital, I was sent home with contact information for rehabilitation therapy. As a side note to my surgery, I only had to stop the Lorlatinib for two days, and Dr. Shaw had asked for all pathology reports from the surgery.

*****

"Live as if you were to die tomorrow. Learn as if you were to live forever." —Mahatma Gandhi

A quote by Mahatma Gandhi that had come to our minds as Connie and I walked the grounds of Gandhi Smriti, the museum dedicated to Gandhi in New Delhi, India, and sadly the site of his assassination in January of 1948. My travels as a person living with terminal lung cancer certainly illustrate my support of Gandhi's philosophy. The Gandhi Museum grounds were a highlight, while the beautiful Taj Mahal (a stopping point on our fast-paced tour of India) was not a reason to visit India, in my humble opinion.

My love for hiking and the mountains led me to include the small country of Nepal in our travels. I was not disappointed. Viewing the 29,035-foot-high Mt. Everest in the Himalayas was absolutely mesmerizing, not to mention the flight landing at the

Kathmandu International airport, which I learned later was known as one of the worst airports in the world. I now understand why. As we circled the airport for a good hour, they began handing out free beer!

An amusing side note was my experience at the New Delhi India airport. To appreciate the following story, it would behoove the reader to hear the following interaction with the Nepal/Indian dialect. As my wife and I were in line at the passport booth, the officer checking passports motioned me to come forward. I handed him my passport, he gave it a good "look-over," looked back at me, back at the passport, and then back at me. As any international traveler will attest, it is not a good sign when the passport official gives the passport and the traveler a second and even third look!

The official stopped the line and then leaned out of his passport booth. He motioned to his cohorts in the booths on both sides to take a look at me. By this time, sweat is running down my back, my wife has this horrified look, and I'm envisioning handcuffs and jail. Now all the other uniformed officials throughout the terminal were looking at me. Actually, it seemed everyone in the airport was looking in my direction! Total quiet for what I thought was an hour, but my wife assured me it was just a minute or so when the official holding my passport yelled out in his broken English for everyone to hear, "Look, George Bush. He look like George Bush!" There was an explosion of laughter throughout the airport as he stamped my passport with a big smile on his face. With the greatest relief, I could not grab that passport fast enough. In doing so, he handed me my passport and, with his ear-to-ear grin, exclaimed, "George Bush Senior!" Connie jokingly suggested that I recheck my genealogy tree when we returned home.

* * * * *

"Hello, Bill. How was your trip to India? Hope you didn't have any gastric gastronomic issues." Now, if you guessed that inquiry could only come from a medical person, you would be correct. Those were the first words out of Dr. Shaw's mouth on her No-

vember 2019 call. She shared that she would soon begin working in research for a drug company; therefore, she would not be
permitted to have patients on clinical trials. I knew the day would
come, even thought about the sad day of not having her as my
oncologist, but every time I pushed that thought to the back of my
mind. Actually, I had read speculation on the ALK Positive website
that she might be moving over to research, so I was not totally unprepared. I appreciated that she was thoughtful and caring
enough to personally call me and share what she was doing and
had arranged for her cohort to take over the clinical trial. Still, I
was sad, for it was Dr. Shaw who literally saved my life and started
me on my ALK journey. Saying she has been amazing does not
seem to be strong enough words. This was the Dr. Shaw; my wife
and I had come to love. A Physician/Oncologist who had an un-
questionable desire to give everything she had to her patients. She
was particularly supportive of all my travels, giving us guidance on
the appropriate precautions due to my low immune system and
the challenges of traveling to foreign countries.

And travel we have! To this point in my cancer journey, we have
traveled the world and then some. This included all seven continents, five Wonders of the World, and visits to all but one of our
63 National Parks.

Oh, the stories we have.

*****

In December 2019, I met Dr. Lin, my new oncologist. My first
visit with Dr. Lin brought a very welcomed change to my blood
thinner medication, both in name brand and application method.
Eliquis in pill form replaced the need for the nasty Arixtra syringe
(needle) to my tender belly. Hard to believe that for five years from
Jan. 2014 to 2019, I was the human pin cushion of the cancer
universe.

As I slunk off the clinic scale on that first visit with Dr. Lin, I
questioned the truthfulness of the scale. I should have anticipated
the dramatic increase in weight, as I had noticed how my midsec-

tion (belly) was getting in the way of the view of my shoes. All this weight gain should not have been a great surprise as I had been warned that Lorlatinib could possibly add 25 pounds. As a matter of fact, it was very likely! Yet the weight increase really bothered me on my visit to MGH. It rocketed to an incredible 215 pounds when I stepped onto the scale! Wow! The most I had ever weighed in my life, let alone the 13-plus years since my cancer diagnosis. I had noticed how my belly, now resembling a bowling ball, had been increasing on Lorlatinib. Knowing my hip replacement resulted in practically no activity; I had expected some weight gain. Yet now, with the weight gain official and a few walks in front of the mirror, reality took hold, and I knew I had to do something. Remembering the extensive discussions on the *ALK-POSITIVE.org* website (a good resource for all dealing with ALK lung cancer) about reducing carbs in the diet, I decided to go with the KETO method. Notice I did not say KETO diet, for I thought I would just read up on the KETO method and, with the help of my home economist wife, go low carb.

As I scanned over an ALK listing of books, one of the entries caught my eye, *"KETO and Cancer."* Surprised to see a book written exclusively on KETO and cancer, I decided to google the two; to my surprise, many books address KETO and cancer. One book's introduction mentioned the importance of being sure to talk with one's oncologist before starting the diet. I had to chuckle to myself. I had not considered that and now realize why my wife was so interested in my blood work results. Duh!

As I mentioned previously, one of the first questions often asked by patients beginning a new clinical trial focused on what side effects to expect. Phase I-II trials, which I have typically been involved with, usually have a list of side effects but caution that there are no absolutes, knowing each patient is different. That said, I have found the side effects they list are usually pretty accurate, and when told on my current trial that I could expect a 25-pound weight gain, it got my attention. After three years on the Lorlatinib trial, I managed to gain 25 pounds and was not a happy camper. About that time, the coronavirus hit, and I became extremely frustrated looking in the mirror and fighting to buckle my pants. I decided to do something about the "bulging belly." Having read a little about the KETO diet, I talked with my wife about possibly cutting my carb intake, and let's see what happens. Well, to my delight, six months later, I was down 35 pounds and had tightened my belt two notches. I could not be happier. Without a doubt, cutting out carbs, and a wife making the greatest meals without the carbs, had done the trick!

Chapter 19
Mask Up!!

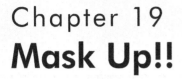

"When you come to the end of your rope,
tie a knot and hang on."
—Franklin D. Roosevelt

* * * * * * * *

What a quandary! COVID 19 in the air, and I'm immunocompromised! A major life change was about to take place for me and many others who were not in any way prepared.

March 2020. I experienced a first as Connie and I prepared for our quarterly trip to Boston for my Lorlatinib clinical trial. A trip that routinely involved a doctor visit, scan review, blood work, EKG, and most importantly, my three-month supply of Lorlatinib. Out of nowhere, I received a call from one of the clinical trial team members who shared that, due to the Corona Virus outbreak, they were recommending I stay home at this time. Wow! What a shocker! Fortunately, I had already sent my brain MRI and chest CT scan results to Boston. So, all they needed would be my blood work completed locally, and they would ship Lorlatinib via FedEx.

Travel plans were no longer necessary when I learned that my Lorlatinib clinical trial hospital visits at MGH were stopped indefinitely. Thankfully, video conferencing with the clinical trial doctor would be an option and pleased to say it turned out to be positive. Although I would have preferred a one-on-one doctor visit, the video option had the time-saving, not to mention the money-saving benefit of not having to travel the 1,700-mile round trip to Boston. A noticeable relief to my wallet!

The phone call from Dr. Lin reassured me that my scans looked good, and I was all set for another three months in the trial. Little did I know how this would evolve, with a few minor adjustments, into a routine for the foreseeable future.

A side note: Knowing the importance of temperature sensitivity and the high cost of Lorlatinib, I was surprised at the willingness of the clinical trial officials to ship my drug. They only asked that I be home to sign and receive the medicine.

COVID-19 had an immediate impact on other travel plans. We had a trip to the Samoa Islands scheduled within the week to visit the last of the 63 National Parks. We were disappointed to cancel the trip but very happy that we would not be captive on a remote island in the South Pacific Ocean with a positive test and quarantined indefinitely! (Update: With covid in the rearview mirror, March 2023 found us visiting National Park number 63, Pago Pago, in the American Samoa Islands.)

The FedEx man delivered; I believe they issued track shoes to the drivers. This thought came from observing the FedEx man who came to the door with my Lorlatinib arm fully extended to hand my wife the package. Even though my wife had her mask on, pen in hand, the very fearful FedEx man was taking no chances of contracting the terrible COVID virus. And we heard him exclaim as he bolted for his truck, "Here's your package, Ma'am, no need for a signature!"

April 2020. Eastern Europe cruise canceled. Ugh!

*****

All good things never last forever. Sadly, Dr. Lin informed me the Lorlatinib trial was closing down, with my next scheduled visit in November to be the last. It had been quite a run, a little over four years since my brain surgery and the beginning of the Lorlatinib trial drug, which had proven so effective that it was fast-tracked and put on the market. So now I had to figure out a way to pay the high monthly cost of Lorlatinib since I would no longer get the drug free of charge from the clinical trial. Bank robbery was not an option, I contacted my insurance, and it looked like they would pay a substantial portion but still leave me with a significant financial burden. Half joking, I told Connie, "There go our travels." We had applied to several agencies for assistance, and I guess the anxiety of waiting for a response was on my mind; hence I often found myself typing on the iPad at four in the morning.

I received some excellent news not long after. My nagging concerns about paying for the cancer drug Lorlatinib had been solved for the time being. More specifically, after being informed that my clinical trial was being shut down and given my last three-month supply of Lorlatinib, Connie and I began checking out other payment options. My clinical trial team gave us numbers to call, along with contact people. As we enjoyed an evening of catching up and comparing ALK notes with friends, we were given a phone number to an individual connected with Pfizer, the company making Lorlatinib.

Connie went to work calling the numbers given to us, which resulted in some great information about the forms Pfizer needed to see what type of financial assistance we could apply for to help cover the cost. As we anxiously awaited to hear from Pfizer, we discussed how our financial situation might become much more of a strain, to put it lightly. Having been informed by my insurance that they would cover a large part of the drug cost, we would still be responsible for several hundred dollars a month, which would likely increase. It looked like our budget would be put to the test as well as our travels, already put to a stop with COVID, could be coming to an end.

The much-anticipated phone call came a week later from a representative of Pfizer, asking to speak to William. I was floored when she nonchalantly informed me of my approval to receive Lorlatinib through Pfizer's Oncology Together program! I could not believe what I was hearing and fumbled to put my cell phone on speaker for Connie to hear as the representative rattled off a few questions, the final being, "When would you like to begin receiving the drug?" I immediately said, "Now." Wow! What a relief! I again asked for details about the program to ensure I heard her correctly. She clarified and said I was approved through December 2020; then, I would have to apply again in January. So, I slept a little easier, knowing that if my health continued, my quality of life would also continue for at least the rest of the year.

*****

October 15, 2020. I haven't given it much thought, but in two days, I would be turning 72. Who would have ever believed I would still be walking this earth, given the devastating stage IV lung cancer diagnosis 13 years ago? Oh, so much has been crammed into those years.

I can say with little hesitance that I had overcome my anxiety about scans, specifically, the MRI scans that required a time of 30 to 40 minutes head-first insertion into a tube. While I am somewhat apprehensive due to past years' experiences, I have recently been able to endure my MRI scans without the mirror. Never thought that would happen. On my last scan for the clinical trial, I asked about the mirror, and a new technician gave me the typical bewildered look, like I had two heads, saying she had no idea where a mask with a mirror would be. While she began to search, I calmly said, "Forget it." To my surprise, I had the scan without concern.

My final clinical trial video conference for the Lorlatinib trial with Dr. Lin and the study team included an in-depth discussion about COVID vaccines. They reinforced my decision to get a vaccine as soon as possible, along with other available boosters. We ended my final study conference with well wishes to all.

*****

Now that my Lorlatinib clinical trial was coming to an end, and my huge relief from learning that Pfizer would provide my medicine. I had not given much thought concerning my doctor. While Dr. Lin had been excellent, with COVID-19 and the lack of face-to-face visits, it wasn't easy to develop the positive vibes I had had with Dr. Shaw.

After some thought, I began to think, "Why not call Dr. Shaw and see if she was possibly taking on a few patients," even though she had begun her work in the area of research. So, I typed a quick email asking about the possibility of me being a patient of hers again. I was pleased to receive an email soon thereafter stating she would be happy to have me as a patient.

Trying to be upfront, I included that I would like to have my scans and visits go from three to four-month intervals and have intermittent doctor visits and video conferences. To my delight, I got a very friendly and affirmative reply. I was thrilled to be again the patient of the doctor who saved my life 13 years ago when I was diagnosed with stage IV inoperable lung cancer. Numerous oncologists and doctors told me in no uncertain terms that I had six months to two years at the most to live.

Nov. 25, 2020. Celebrating our 50th wedding anniversary with a trip in our Argosy travel trailer to the newest of the National Parks. White Sands in New Mexico was a great getaway from all the anxiety of COVID. Who would have guessed that with my stage IV cancer diagnosis in 2007, I would be around to celebrate 50 years of marriage? An interesting fact I came across is that only 6 percent of married couples reach their golden anniversary. What a milestone!

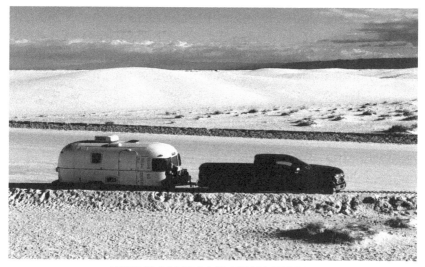

WHITE SANDS NP, NEW MEXICO

✵ ✵ ✵ ✵ ✵

January 2021. A video conference with Dr. Shaw was planned as my first since leaving the clinical trial. Back together, albeit not in person, a phone conversation with Dr. Shaw was certainly a reassuring moment in my cancer journey. We had planned for a video teleconference, but that didn't work, so Dr. Shaw called me at the scheduled time and reviewed my CT & MRI scans. I must say it was comforting knowing that Dr. Shaw was "back in my corner" for my continued lung cancer fight. It had been well over a year since Dr. Shaw shared that she would enter a more in-depth research position associated with a drug company and, therefore, would not be directly involved with clinical trial patients. With my clinical trial days behind me, I was again able to have Dr. Shaw as my oncologist, and I could not be happier. Knowing that my cancer future would continue to evolve, there is no one else I would want on my cancer journey.

* * * * *

Great news! I received the long-awaited call from Pfizer again approving my application to receive their drug Lorbrena (Lorlatinib) for the following calendar year. Difficult to express the relief, knowing that at least for another year, I would not have to worry about finding a way to pay the very high cost.

Now, if we could only hear from our county health department about the COVID-19 vaccine we were scheduled to receive in the next couple of weeks, the anxiety of waiting would be over for a while. Interestingly, one of the vaccine drugs is also produced by Pfizer.

The mad search for drugs. One would think Connie and I were drug junkies looking for a fix rather than just a couple of old fogies looking to get our first of two COVID-19 vaccine shots. It had been somewhat challenging, to say the least. We were told by the State of Ohio, in charge of getting the vaccine out to Ohio residents, to sign up at our local health department and wait until our age group, 70-and-above, was called. The major quandary was the lack of the drug allocated to Ohio and not hearing any information from our local health department. After seeing on Facebook that the medication was being dispensed at other locations and available to whoever signed up, Connie was able to go online and schedule our vaccine shots at a CVS facility.

Our two Pfizer vaccine shots were finally history; we had heard the two shots taken two weeks apart would be approximately 95 percent effective at the end of two weeks. So, hopefully, we could get on with our lives without the suffocating mask! Although the governor had not lifted the mask mandate, other states had; hopefully, as the COVID cases declined, Ohio residents would also be free of the COVID restrictions.

*****

The possibility of cancer returning is always in the back of an individual's mind. Below is an excellent article by Jeffery Sturm that I believe shares the feelings of many living with cancer:

HI Folks. Here's the follow-up post to my last one from my Facebook page. It's one of a series I've been running since early 2015.

Carcinoma Commentaries

3/6/2021

Complete Response

These were the first two words on the PET scan report handed to me this week, evidencing the success of the new drug I've been on for two months to address a recurrence of lung cancer. They were followed by the words "no evidence of disease", and then a lot of other information about absent tumors and quiescent lymph nodes. Metastatic lung cancer. Erased. In two months. Think about it.

The cancer is not dead however; it's only been put to sleep. There is no cure as yet, and it could wake up at any time. Six years after original diagnosis, we've managed to suppress it again in my body with a much stronger, more tolerable drug. But lung cancer is ingenious. It will find a way to mutate around the drug in time, and return in a more virulent form. We're not ready for that demon yet, but the researchers are hard at it. There are thousands of people like me, still alive, doing time, waiting for the next scan, blood test, verdict, clinical trial. In-between.

That oh-so-valuable time in-between. Someone hands you a piece of paper that says you're going to live. The shadowy thumb of fate emerges from the mist, pointed skyward. The proverbial parachute snaps open and the deepest possible silence accompanies your freefall to a gentle landing on a planet you've never seen so clearly before. Everything is new, beautiful, precious. The simple pleasure of having the time to enjoy life for a while seems beyond all valuation, an immeasurable gift. The overwhelmingly exquisite rush of love for life itself, for the effortless joy of being human and possessing some time to savor that privilege. The profound relief at the dissipation of pain and fragility. And at the heart of it, gratitude.

Gratitude like a current, flowing out to friends and family, loved ones and supporters who have buoyed Ellen and me through the many stages of both our cancer ordeals for a decade. Gratitude to the ALK+ community members on Facebook who support each other through the day-to-day in-betweens, share information, and provide guidance in the face of mortal uncertainty. Gratitude to the small community of ALK clinicians and researchers at the teaching hospitals and pharmaceutical companies for their tireless dedication to saving our lives. Gratitude to the oncology docs and staff whose persistent expertise and kindness make the treatments livable.

And deep humility for the fact that I'm doing well, when so many others are not, or have passed. Something like 1,800,000 people die every year from lung cancer, over 150,000 of them in the U.S. ALK+ Non-Small Cell Adenocarcinoma of the Lung, or ALK+ NS-CLC, occurs in about 3-5% of lung cancer patients, the vast majority of whom were never smokers. It can strike at any age; cause unknown. When I was diagnosed in 2014, if the first of the ALK+ drugs had not been available, my life expectancy was six months. If that.

Humility indeed, and prayers. Jubilation for another day.

*****

On the road again. This time a visit with my youngest son and family in sunny California via our travel trailer. A flood of memories returned as I thought about a similar California trip 12 years earlier. The difference being in the earlier trip, my thoughts centered around the fact that I was dying, and it would be doubtful I would ever return to California for a visit. It was especially difficult knowing, in all likelihood, it would be the last time to ever see my son and his family. I was at that time headed to California awaiting news from Dr. Shaw about my 3 to 5 percent chance of qualifying for a possible last-chance, life-saving clinical trial.

Oh, how things have changed. Now, 12 years later, I was driving to California for a night in the mountains with a crew of rookie smokejumpers that my son was training. Sitting around a campfire in the Northern California mountains with a group of young men wrapping up a tough two months of training was indeed enlightening, to say the least. Although I must admit, the rock digging into my backside throughout the night made my 72-year-old body ready for a warm, soft bed.

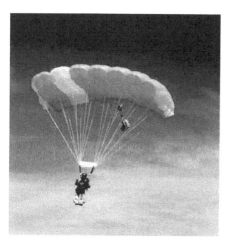 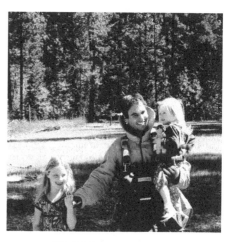

BRAD,
SMOKEJUMPER TRAINING

GRANDDAUGHTERS
HAPPY TO SEE DAD

The following day, after a night spent under the stars with the smokejumpers, I was sitting at my son's dining room table in Redding, California, having a video conference with Dr. Shaw. What a wonderful opportunity modern technology had availed me as I was able to video conference while on vacation. The only negative was that during the conference, Dr. Shaw informed me that out-of-state video conferences would no longer be permissible due to hospital rules. What a shame! Technology finally caught up with patient-doctor communication needs, and they suspended its use! Why?

My health is "stable," the word I had come to live with since my cancer journey began some 13 years ago when told the word "Stable" is what the doctors and I wanted to see. "Stable" basically means no progress in my cancer.

Sadly, a fellow patient living with lung cancer was not dealing with 'stable." This was not just any fellow patient, but rather the individual I first saw on TV those 12 years ago. One of the first ALK patients of Dr. Shaw, who said on network news her cancer was "melting away" and which offered me my first flicker of hope. That individual, Linnea, was literally fighting for her life. Linnea, the epitome of the cancer "fighting warrior."

Never in my wildest dreams did I ever believe I would become complacent about my lung cancer? There had been many times throughout my cancer journey when I thought back to my times of excellent health and wondered if I would ever feel that good again. I do now and can't believe I had become complacent. It doesn't take, but a quick read of Linnea's blog, and I am returned to reality. My cancer is still with me, but thanks to the incredible Dr. Shaw and all the nurse practitioners and their associates, it remains "stable" at this time.

* * * * *

Another set of scans at the Upper Valley Medical Center. My routine of scans had undoubtedly made some changes since my first scans some 13-14 years ago. First, the challenges I had with claustrophobia and the dreadful "machine from hell," the MRI Machine! That terrible claustrophobic experience subsided with time, but I am unsure why. With my fingers crossed, my most recent MRI scan, usually dreaded for days in advance, basically was a walk in the park. No more calling ahead to make sure I was scheduled for the largest machine or requesting the face mask with the attached mirror enabling me to see outside the tube. Now, after well over 100 scans, it was simply a part of my life, a bump in the road, so to speak.

The other change with scans, both the MRI and CAT, was the reporting process. A few years back, the wait time for scan results was maddening, the common practice of the scan results being sent to the doctor and not directly to the patient compounded the wait. Anyone who has ever been in the situation of waiting to hear about the result of their scans knows the anguish of the wait. All that changed, at least for me, as I shared with a couple of friends while discussing the anxiety of waiting for scan results. I had completed both an MRI / CAT scan the day before, and I already had my scan results. The hospital had emailed my results and a very detailed report completed by a resident physician that same day. I can't begin to verbalize the relief of reading a report that described, "stable" and the relaxed feeling it gave me on the long ride to Boston. Of course, at my visit with Dr. Shaw, we would again discuss the results of my scans, and I would be able to ask questions, but the relief of knowing the results of the scans immediately was tremendous.

*****

September 2021. Big news. Wow! What a day I had, maybe one of the best in my cancer journey! I finally returned to MGH in Boston and had a face-to-face conference with Dr. Shaw. Due to COVID, it was the first conference in over two years! As mentioned previously, she had moved on to more involvement in the research aspect of cancer while keeping a few patients on Thursday visits at the hospital. Because she had gone into research, she was no longer able to work with clinical trial patients. With my clinical trial coming to an end, I was able to hook up with her again; hence our meeting. After catching up on the past couple of years, we discussed the blood work and scans I had FedEx-ed to her.

Everything looked normal, and she did not see any reason for a change. Then as we began discussing both the MRI and CAT scans, she threw me the big changeup, saying the scans both looked good and she would recommend extending the time between the scans to six months. I just about fell off the exam table I was sitting on! I had requested to extend the time between scans at every conference over the years without much success. Ecstatic, yet apprehensive! Thinking back, I probably should have discussed the move to six months with Dr. Shaw in a little more detail.

*****

October 5, 2021. Now that was a surprise. I walked into the dentist's office for a second opinion on a decaying tooth and minutes later walked out without the aforementioned tooth! Not that I did not want the tooth removal to take place; I was just not expecting the dentist to do it right after advising me the tooth needed to come out. Actually, I was more than happy to have the extraction completed in such a timely manner.

Could my cancer have been the cause? Tooth absorption decay is what Dr. Davis called my need for the tooth extraction. "Cause?" This is always the question of a person living with cancer when confronted with a new medical occurrence. "Nope, it just happens," was his reply.

Chapter 20
"Miles to Go Before I Sleep"

"Sometimes even to live is an act of courage."
–Lucius Annaeus Seneca

* * * * * * * *

Celebrated my 73rd birthday with a maiden voyage in our new-to-us travel trailer. Connie and I traveled to Punderson State Park east of Cleveland, just a few miles from my sister and brother-in-law's home. A delightful two-day vacation. We got to catch up on what was happening in their lives: kids, health, oh yeah, always the health. The old saying, "It's hell to get old, but the alternative is worse," is so true. Our visit took me back to my earliest cancer days when I received the devastating stage IV terminal cancer diagnosis at the Cleveland Clinic. Words cannot express my appreciation for my sister and her husband, as they offered all the hospitality we could have imagined. I believe all my fellow cancer warriors echo my sentiments regarding the importance of assistance from others. I noted this in the Cancer & Friends chapter of my book.

Connie and I anxiously awaited opportunities to travel again with plans to visit the grandkids in New York. Hopefully, the COVID vaccine will "deep six" many of our concerns. Our Eastern Europe River cruise with Viking, which we had scheduled the past year with the hope COVID-19 issues would be behind us, had been canceled. We now rebooked on an ocean cruise called the Journey to Antiquities, from Rome to Athens, for November, trusting all travel restrictions would be lifted by then. Viking River Cruise Line had informed us that they had instituted some very stringent rules regarding COVID restrictions and had invested in robot-like characters roaming the hallways and public spaces cleaning and disinfecting during the late-night hours. I smiled to myself at the thought of a somewhat inebriated passenger weaving his way through the corridor on his way to his stateroom and suddenly coming face-to-face with a junior E.T.!

It seems like a birthday typically brings many memories of the past, as likely experienced by other individuals living with cancer. A flood of faces and many friendships are etched in my mind. Sadly, my thoughts also are of so many who are no longer with us, which reminds me how fortunate I am to still be here.

Enough of the morbid talk. We are looking forward to our next big adventure, an ocean cruise in Europe. It's been a while in the making with the challenges of COVID still "lingering" in our midst, with the different strains constantly evolving. Too many deaths are still happening! I've taken the vaccines and was first in line for the booster shot, deciding some time ago that I would not stop my travel plans and life, if at all possible.

*****

Nov. 15, 2021. A very sad day. I just read a post by her daughter on Facebook that Linnea Olson had passed away. Twelve years ago, early in my struggle with lung cancer and after approximately two years of ineffective chemo combinations that brought me to my knees and death's door, I met Linnea via ABC National News. Lying on my couch, unable to physically climb the stairs, up popped Linnea on a national news broadcast from a cancer seminar in Florida. Her words echo through my mind 12 years later, "I have stage IV adenocarcinoma, and it is melting away!" Those words led me to Dr. Shaw and MGH.

It was on the seventh floor of the Yawkey Center for Cancer Care at MGH. I was just finishing a meeting with Dr. Alice Shaw, who was in the early days of an ALK clinical trial, Crizotinib. One of Dr. Shaw's first ALK patients, Linnea, sat in the waiting room. I was certainly encouraged to see a very positive and vibrant early ALK patient doing so well. After that, Linnea and I met in passing on a few other occasions. A cancer kinship evolved as I followed her progress through her very personal and informative blog. I must admit my close following was essentially a personal desire to see her succeed, knowing/hoping my health would continue to be positive. I say in all sincerity, truly rest in peace, ALK Warrior Linnea.

*****

We received some challenging news. As I have previously mentioned, I had been very fortunate to have received Lorbrena from Pfizer's patient assistance program for the last two years. Each December involved a new application that included medical and financial information. Considering nothing had changed, we had hoped the assistance would continue without interruption. That was not the case; they had requested we apply to three specific organizations and get back to them on what was offered. More hoops to jump through! We immediately contacted the three organizations and were told we did not qualify for any of the three; two were not even taking applications at that time. So having informed Pfizer of our inability to get assistance from the three organizations they requested we contact, it was a fingers-crossed wait.

*****

February 2022. I was done with clinical trials. At least, I hoped so! While reminiscing about all our travels to Boston for the three previous clinical trials, I asked Connie to look up the number of trips (round trip 1700 miles) we had taken to Boston. I thought the number was high, but I was surprised when she said 92! And get this, 49 MRIs and 89 CTs. That was only after I began going to Boston. Not counted were the MRI/CT scans the first two years following diagnosis, before the first clinical trial in Boston. So now we all know why I can light up a dark room when entering without turning on the lights! A side note, I remember when first discussing my cancer and concern over the high number of scans I was required to undergo with Dr. Shaw, she simply stated, "Bill, that is the least of your worries!" Wonder what she would say now. Maybe I'll ask her at our next conference.

An interesting tidbit from the scan tech I had talked with after my recent six-month scan; notice I said six months. What a blessing and wonderful reprieve from the maddening three-month scan schedule I had for years. I digress. I asked a question I had been wondering about for over 16 years whenever I had my first MRI, a question I believe any occupant of the "tube" had at some time throughout their ordeal. As the technician slowly slid me out of the MRI machine like a loaf of bread, I asked, "Why do those MRI machines have to make such a loud noise?" He answered, "The gradient." My look of puzzlement was sadly matched by his difficulty finding further words of explanation. So, at home, I referred to Google and found the cause for the noise of the MRI:

> *"The Gradient magnetic field is the main source of acoustic noise associated with an MRI procedure. This noise occurs during the rapid alterations of currents within the gradient coils."*

So, there you have it. Now you know why one should never turn down the offer of a headset and your favorite music when entering the "tube!"

* * * * *

Having not heard from Pfizer, I called and was overjoyed to learn that I was approved for another year. Quite the relief!!

Very high on the "concern scale" of all individuals living with cancer is that of finance, specifically that of paying the very high cost of drugs, scans, and other medical procedures. In the case of drugs, at the time of this writing, I was on the very expensive Lorlatinib. Connie and I previously shared the very involved process we had to go through with Pfizer, which was obviously very beneficial in getting assistance for the drug.

* * * * *

I woke up in a cold sweat, not the first time, actually an occasional occurrence. Wondering if it was cancer-related? Wondering why I am just now wondering! I guess I had other issues more concerning than a little sweat. Not sure if I have ever heard other patients mention occasional cold sweat occurrences.

I had some really tired legs yesterday on my hike to the Prairie. Cancer related? Maybe. Or was it the ordeal I dealt with after my scans yesterday? I had a serious bout with diarrhea that had me making a quick pit stop on our drive home from the hospital. All these questions! Oh, the life of a person living with cancer. Yes, I know, better than the alternative.

*****

Did I mention it never ends?

One of the challenges I had dealt with off and on since my cancer diagnosis was the various minor ailments, always wondering if they were cancer related. An example was the current issue involving eye floaters, which I believe some call "nets." I describe them as "spider webs" floating around in the corner of my left eye. I had them off and on over the years. They seemed to become a bit more prevalent and especially irritating with the accompanying light flashes when out in the sunlight.

Having experienced floaters previously and sharing the occurrence with my optometrist at my yearly checkup, he had indicated it was not too concerning. But somewhat age-related, and I would simply need to keep a proverbial "eye" on it.

After my daily "old man's morning workout" (25 pushups and 25 squat thrusts), I noticed a return of some floaters in my vision that, throughout the day, evolved into some flashing lights, including darkness and cloudiness.

Of course, the eye floater had to worsen at the end of the day, on Friday of Super Bowl weekend! Therefore, I thought it reasonable to wait until the following Monday to arrange a visit with my local optometrist, a decision I would come to regret.

I called the optometrist's office first thing Monday morning and was told they were booked solid. Could I wait until the following day? Grudgingly, I scheduled an appointment for the next day. Minutes later, I got a call from the optometrist telling me to get over to his office immediately; he would work me in. Within minutes I was in the exam room, where my optometrist detected a detached retina and was making arrangements for surgery the next day. Thank the good Lord for small-town personal care!

The following day I found myself flat on my back on the surgery table. Obviously, time was a concern; and having been several days since I first noticed the symptoms, it was essential to reattach my retina expeditiously.

The morning following my eye surgery. What the hell happened?

I awoke and rolled over on my back to see the time, a very blurry 3:39 a.m. My wife quietly reminded me I had had surgery and the doctor's orders were not to sleep on my back.

It all was starting to come back to me as I climbed out of bed, feeling my way to the bathroom. There I glanced weary-eyed into the mirror. I was stunned at the sight of all the bandages, or an even more explicit description would be that of a wounded WW I soldier looking back at me. The enormous gauze and tape bandage over my left eye began to revive my memory of the previous 24 hours of torment I had undergone.

On the second day following my detached retina surgery, a follow-up visit with the optometrist assured me that all had gone well with the surgery. He felt confident that my eyesight would gradually improve throughout the week.

Since I had been told to limit most activities, the downtime had given me a lot of time to think. During my first meeting with the optometrist and discussing the diagnosis of a detached retina, I shared my cancer experience and asked if there was any connection. He assured me there was no connection between the two, that a detached retina can "just happen."

I found that somewhat unique, for I think back when I asked the cause of my lung cancer, stating I had never smoked and received the same response: lung cancer could "just happen!"

*****

A new man to the fight. I just turned another page in my lung cancer journey by introducing a new doctor to my team of ALK-gifted warriors in my 16-year-old cancer battle. With the recommendation of Dr. Shaw and a change in my scan schedule to six-month intervals, I was now seeing another oncologist. We arranged to see Dr. Shaw in Boston and a local doctor at six-month intervals. It would involve sending a copy of the scan report to Dr. Shaw for her review and, at the same time, conferring with the local doctor to discuss my scans and blood work and answer any questions I might have.

The local oncologist, Dr. Joseph Lavelle, was recommended by Dr. Shaw and fellow local ALK patient Jeff Meckstroth and his wife Rhonda as being very knowledgeable about ALK. I could not have been more pleased with their recommendation. On our first visit, I found Dr. Lavelle well-versed in ALK and very personable. I was especially impressed that he had taken the time to read through all my background paperwork the previous night at his home and seemed excited to be working with me as his patient. I was also surprised and reassured that he currently had four other ALK patients.

What definitely sealed the deal on my positive opinion of Dr. Lavelle was toward the end of our conversation when he casually mentioned he did not ask his patients to drink the putrid contrast before scans. Now that was a doctor after my own heart! I had been one of those pathetic individuals required to somehow gulp down the horrible dried-concrete-like substance.

* * * * *

278 days until we cast off from the port in Athens for a Journey to Antiquities cruise aboard the Viking ship Sky. This would be the fourth try on a cruise in the last two years; all previously canceled trips had been due to that nasty COVID! To say COVID had put a crimp in our travel plans would be putting it mildly. There was a time when putting off travel plans was not a major issue, but having a stage IV terminal cancer diagnosis highlighted the need for a bit of urgency in future plans!

* * * * *

A little levity on my next follow-up visit with the eye surgeon, I met with an assistant who began with a straightforward hand check of my vision by first covering my good eye. She then placed some fingers in front of my repaired eye and asked the number, to which I quickly replied, "Fingers? I can't even see your hand!" I heard a very faint, almost inaudible, "Oh my," as she left the room.

Yikes! I could not see anything; my left eye was still blurry. As the doctor calmly began the exam, he indicated he was expecting better vision. He decided on an ultrasound to ensure my retina was attached correctly. Finding my retina was indeed attached, he suggested, "It's just blood." Guess another side effect of blood thinners when you are living with cancer.

April 8, 2022. Milestone! 15 years ago, this date marked my official diagnosis of stage IV Lung Cancer. Needless to say, a date that absolutely changed my life forever.

*****

Connie and I had an enjoyable visit and dinner with two wonderful new friends, Jeff and Rhonda Meckstroth. We happened to meet through our mutual ALK lung cancer journey.

Jeff, a quiet-spoken retired farmer and firefighter was diagnosed with stage IV lung cancer in 2015. As so often, his cancer was discovered during a routine annual physical with his primary care physician after mentioning a lingering, non-productive cough.

Rhonda, who I soon learned to be quite the cancer warrior, was a true advocate for her husband. She learned in 2017 that I had stage IV lung cancer and contacted me through the ALK Positive website. I could tell by her message the lady was on a mission and was looking for something positive for her husband's cancer. Rhonda proceeded to tell me that Jeff was currently seeing an oncologist that had recommended Whole Brain Radiation for his brain Mets.

Fortunately, she had heard of Dr. Shaw, emailed her for advice, and received a resounding, "Don't do Whole Brain Radiation!" Having learned I currently was one of Dr. Shaw's patients, she reached out to me and asked if we could meet to talk. I happily invited Rhonda and Jeff over to our home in Versailles. As the four of us discussed where Jeff was in his treatment plan, it became very obvious that Whole Brain Radiation had been put on the pro-verbial back burner. I'm pleased to share that the following years have seen our friendship continue to grow with backyard visits, as well as breakfast and lunch get-togethers.

An interesting side note and find: When I went to investigate more information about Lorbrena, I naturally did an internet search. To my surprise and great pleasure, a Google search took me to a Lorbrena page with my very good friends Jeff and Rhonda Meckstroth smiling back at me on the front page.

As our visits with Jeff and Rhonda continued, chats on the advancement in ALK lung cancer were always front and center. This includes the current research into a fourth-generation "double mutant active" ALK TKIs such as Gilteritinib, TPX-0131, and NVL-655. Hurrah for research!! This is certainly exciting news for all ALK Patients.

*****

I returned from a nice walk uptown to our local friendly drug store for a Moderna COVID booster. After talking with both on-cologists, Dr. Shaw and Dr. Lavelle, I was assured that it would be vital for me, living with lung cancer, stage IV and immunocompro-mised, to receive the booster. Since I previously had three Pfizer vaccines, it was the opinion of the doctors and the pharmacist that I consider a change to Moderna, because it could be more effec-tive in controlling the current virus making the rounds.

We planned to travel across the country (of course, using our travel trailer) following the Oregon Trail in a few weeks, so we fig-ured it best to have the booster several weeks beforehand to make sure we were not on the road with some type of reaction. They sure have made it easy for an elderly 73-year-old living with terminal lung cancer to get a COVID booster.

Wow! Wow! Wow! Nothing like a triple wow to express the impact of the Moderna vaccine drug on Connie and me. To say it kicked our butts would be putting it mildly. We felt pretty good the first evening, to the point that we even took a bike ride out of town to visit friends. But a reaction became apparent throughout the night, as Connie and I both had difficulty sleeping; due to a sore, inflamed arm and headache. The next morning, we were both still wiped out. I believe we certainly made the right decision getting the Moderna drug early rather than closer to heading West on our trip along the Oregon Trail. A splitting headache became the norm, along with some major sofa time throughout the day for both Connie and me.

Two days later, we both were doing just fine. Guess we both were a bit surprised by our reaction to the Moderna COVID Vaccine, remembering how Pfizer seemed more amiable to our aging, mellowing bodies.

* * * * *

At 4:20 a.m., I awoke unable to sleep with a throbbing in my upper left leg. I had gone to bed with a sore leg but was unsure what that was all about. Once again, the unknown. So much of living with lung cancer, and I would imagine any cancer, is not knowing why certain things are happening to your body. Then throw in the unique elements of a clinical trial, and you are testing the waters of the unknown. I would like to have a dollar for every time I asked my doctors "Why" and was simply told they didn't know. "You are the first person to experience that issue." And please remember, I had the most intelligent doctors in the world!

* * * * *

At this point, please allow me a few words on three letters, "NED" (no evidence of disease). As discussed early on in this book, my focus and energy had centered on the very positive theme of hope, in which I viewed lung cancer as a disease to live with and not necessarily a curable disease. It is a difficult concept to wrap one's head around, but as I quickly discovered, the sooner I accepted lung cancer as a part of my life, the sooner I could get on with living. I also came to learn early on that I did not need to be NED to get on with my life and live out my dreams to the fullest. I believe that if one checked this book's previous chapters, one would not find the letters NED anywhere within. Probably not the case in the many books on cancer one would typically come across, and it doesn't seem to matter if the site is a reputable one or a site of voodoo and magical concoctions. While I'm well aware of the use of NED in the different articles, blogs, and websites often visited by many individuals living with cancer, NED is simply not part of my vocabulary or, for that matter, my world. I would venture that the main reason I do not use NED is due to the fact I seldom heard it used by Dr. Shaw or, for that matter, any doctors, nurses, or medical personnel that I had the occasion to visit. When taking the time to look back and think about it, I don't remember NED being used within the entire health community I have been involved with over the years.

In no way do I mean to disparage anyone for their use of the term. To be honest, I can't think of a better, more hopeful four words to utter than "No Evidence of Disease." With no offense meant to anyone, I am unsure if there is a more ambiguous phrase than "no evidence of disease." The basis for the aforementioned assertion is from practical observation and hearing the proclamation so often of being NED, followed sadly by the dreaded recurrence of cancer. I find myself wincing when I hear the phrase being used, for I believe it gives false hope. While I certainly believe in hope (I'm all about hope), I believe it imperative that a person living with cancer should always be prepared to "manage" their cancer rather than believe it will go away and stay away. A patient must remain vigilant to the possibility cancer may come back and see to it that it is monitored regularly. I don't believe there was ever a time when this was truer than now. With the advent of all the new TKIs being researched and approved. Now that I have that off my chest, I'll finish with another phrase that has me scratching my head along with "No Evidence of Disease:" "I'm cured." Need I say more?

"I've changed my mindset. I'm not "chasing NED" anymore. NED comes and goes. NED causes anxiety. Like a Jack-in-the-Box, NED makes you anxiously wait for the next 'bad scan.'Nope, I'm not chasing NED. I'm chasing CURE!"
—Alkies Unlimited Danielle Paul James
Fri. May 13, 2022

* * * * *

While my book may come to a close, the battle of living with cancer continues. With this in mind, I have listed Sources and Suggestions along with a recommendation to join the ALK Positive Facebook support group. Being a member of the ALK Positive site on Facebook has undoubtedly enabled me to keep abreast of my many ALK cohorts, not only in the United States but literally worldwide.

I have a particular affinity for the ALK Positive website, as I was immediately attracted to the site when it originated in 2015 by Merita Carroll and her husband, Thomas. It is a sad story, yet it shows that sometimes out of tragedy comes something special, as in the case of Merita and her battle with cancer. Merita was living with stage IV ALK Positive lung cancer and looking for a support community to share information. Sadly, she passed away in 2018. Nonetheless, the ALK Positive community Merita and Thomas started has blossomed into a great source of information for thousands of ALK patients and caregivers worldwide.

* * * * *

There has been some talk in the cancer community regarding "weeding the garden," a phrase associated with Dr. Ross Camidge. Following are my light-hearted thoughts on weeds in a garden.

For years you have worked in your garden (life), laying out seeds that begin to grow in nice neat rows (going to school, learning skills that help you in life), and then someone (cancer) comes along out of nowhere with a large rake and wreaks havoc throughout your garden. Messing up all the nice neat rows (life's plans) you have planted that were beginning to grow and mature. Devastated, all you want to do is sit down and cry. Friends and loved ones come by and sympathize with you, offering words of hope and encouragement but no real answers on how you can restore your plants (life) that you have worked so hard to see grow to maturity. Then, out of nowhere, a glimmer of hope, just when you thought there was no hope for your garden (life) along comes a smiling stranger (oncologist) carrying a big rake (ALK-Positive). With no guarantee of saving your garden (life), the stranger begins to rake your garden, reviving some of your plants (offering a bit of hope) that, indeed, one can live with lung cancer.

National Lung Cancer Awareness Month. I cannot think of a better time than National Lung Cancer Awareness Month to bring my book to a close. While I bring my book to a conclusion, my cancer sojourn continues. It is with sadness that I end my book, knowing all books must come to an end yet knowing full well my story is far from over. Trusting, believing I have many more days of life and adventure ahead. How much longer? I, as well as all my fellow members of the cancer community, ask this question as we travel our separate journeys of "Living with Terminal Lung Cancer".

**"I live life to the fullest each and every day.
That is what sustains me through my journey
of living with cancer."**

—William G. Schuette

Sources
and
Suggestions

"Cancer is messy and scary.
You throw everything at it,
but don't forget to throw love at it.
It turns out that might be the best weapon of all."
—Regina Brett

* * * * * * * *

Throughout my 16-plus years of living with and managing my cancer. I have come across many sources that have been beneficial and hopefully useful for any cancer community members. As for sources of information, there are books, magazines, and websites by the score that one can use for information on the various cancers, both specific and non-specific. Some sources you may want to scrutinize very closely. As I shared earlier, how many well-meaning friends offered advice along with their unique remedies. Please note I said "well-meaning friends." One should know that the unique remedies from an occasional friend are not your primary concern, nor are the back page advertisements in a Sunday morning magazine selling the "sure cure" pills, which will purge your body of all ills in the next 24 hours. No, surprisingly, I'm going to suggest you begin your scrutiny with a very unlikely individual: your doctor, the individual most patients turn to when first diagnosed with cancer. Choosing the correct doctor is one of the most critical decisions a newly-diagnosed patient has to make. A thorough investigation of doctors/oncologists and hospitals must be completed; I cannot overly express the importance. And, of course, the big red flag! If your diagnosing doctor wants to immediately begin using some type of chemotherapy before genetic testing (Genomic Testing), run, don't walk out that door! There may be exceptions to what I just said, for I am not a doctor. Still, I certainly caution any individual to question any immediate chemotherapy before genetic testing, particularly if it involves lung cancer.

Due to having been one of Dr. Shaw's early ALK-positive patients, I have been asked to share my story on various national newscasts, resulting in many people contacting me for information and advice. The first thing I noticed when talking with newly-diagnosed patients living with cancer was the seemingly large number who were unaware of genetic testing and were immediately ushered into the chemotherapy rooms for infusions. Thus, my first question to all newly-diagnosed patients was, "Have you had a biopsy?" followed up with, "Have you had it genetically tested?"

If either answer was no, my immediate comment was, "Run, don't walk, to a doctor/oncologist/hospital that will perform the genetic testing (Genomic Testing) immediately."

In essence, I strongly suggest beginning your research for a medical team at a well-known cancer research hospital, preferably specific to your type of cancer. This can all be done by a search on the internet. After finding a research hospital you are comfortable with, be a sponge and read every bit of information you can find. Ask your doctor for resources.

Over the previous 16-plus years, I have seen the development of many websites created specifically for various cancers. These sites are numerous and sometimes seem overwhelming, so I suggest monitoring two or three to see if one fits your needs and type of cancer.

For general cancer questions and comments, I have been a member of the website *Inspire.com* for many years and while mainly a lurker, I have found the daily bulletins very informative. While a rather large website, I found searching within Inspire.com enabled me to find a group discussion centered on my specific lung cancer.

Regarding resources, there is a website that assists people with locating a biomarker support group for their lung cancer:

https://biomarkercollaborative.org/find-your-group/

A few of the website support groups I am currently monitoring include:

ALK-POSITIVE.org

ALKies Unlimited, and

Lungevity.org.

The following YouTube site is a wonderful source for patients and caregivers promoting ALK-positive cancer awareness and the latest research findings:

https://www.youtube.com/c/ALKLungCancer

INDEX

W

Made in USA - Kendallville, IN
27692_9798988063018
11.06.2023 1308